RAGHURAM'S OCCUPATIONAL THERAPY

- THE HANDWRITING REVOLUTION -
SCRIBBLE TO SCRIPT

RAGHURAM PATTUSAMY

Co-Authors: Jose Mary Sangeetha X,
Loganathan S & T. Sundaresan

notionpress
.com

INDIA · SINGAPORE · MALAYSIA

ISBN 979-8-89446-319-3

Dedicated to

My late parents

Thiru. N. Pattusamy and Thirumathi. K. Poongavanam

&

My brother **Thiru. N. P. Vetri Kulasekaran**

who has been my inspiration and the

driving force for all my accomplishments

in both personal and professional life.

With the Blessings of

Founder Chancellor: Shri. N.P.V Ramasamy Udayar
Chancellor: Thiru. V. R. Venkataachalam
Pro Chancellor: Thiru. R.V. Sengutuvan

HELPING SMALL HANDS MAKE BIG MOVES

AN OCCUPATIONAL THERAPIST TRANSFORMS SCRIBBLES INTO LEGIBLE SCRIPT

CONTENTS

FOREWORD

I am deeply honoured and delighted to write this foreword for "Raghuram's Occupational Therapy - The Handwriting Revolution: Scribble to Script."

Handwriting is a fundamental skill that profoundly impacts various aspects of our lives, from academic achievement to professional success. For individuals undergoing Occupational Therapy, mastering handwriting can be a pivotal milestone in their journey toward independence and an enhanced quality of life. The ability to write legibly and effectively not only supports educational and career opportunities but also fosters self-confidence and personal expression.

In this comprehensive book, the intricacies of handwriting are meticulously explored through the lens of Occupational Therapy. The author has crafted a resource that is both informative and practical, demonstrating a deep understanding of the complexities involved. This book stands out for its thorough approach, combining theoretical insights with actionable strategies that can be applied in various therapeutic contexts.

Occupational Therapy practitioners play a crucial role in facilitating handwriting development and remediation for individuals with handwriting difficulties. Through structured interventions and treatment strategies, Occupational Therapists empower their clients to overcome obstacles and achieve their handwriting goals. This book provides valuable guidance on these interventions, making it an indispensable tool for practitioners dedicated to enhancing their clients' handwriting skills.

Moreover, this book serves as a valuable guide for Occupational Therapists, educators, students, and caregivers seeking to support individuals of all ages in improving their handwriting skills. It offers a wealth of knowledge and practical advice that can be applied in clinical settings, educational environments, and at home, ensuring that individuals receive the comprehensive support they need to succeed.

Beyond its functional utility, this book underscores the broader significance of handwriting. It recognizes handwriting as a form of self-expression, creativity, and cognitive engagement, highlighting its therapeutic benefits for mental well-being and holistic development. Handwriting is more than a motor skill; it is a gateway to cognitive and emotional growth, providing individuals with a medium to communicate their thoughts, ideas, and emotions.

Let us celebrate the achievements, both big and small, that arise from the dedicated efforts of Occupational Therapists. Their work in developing and refining handwriting skills is not only about improving functional capabilities but also about enriching lives and fostering a sense of accomplishment and self-worth.

I commend the author for his dedication to advancing the field of Occupational Therapy and for providing a valuable resource that will undoubtedly inspire and empower Occupational Therapy practitioners worldwide. This book is a testament to the importance of specialized knowledge and the impact of dedicated practice in transforming lives.

May this book inspire readers to embrace the journey toward wholeness with courage, compassion, and unwavering resolve.

With warm regards,

Dr. Pankaj Bajpai (OT)
President-AIOTA (2024-2028)
Former Associate Professor & Head
Dept. of Occupational Therapy, NILD (DEPwD,MSJE,GOI),
Kolkata, West Bengal, India
Former Director (Offg.), NILD, Kolkata, West Bengal, India
Former Dy. Director Administration (Offg.), NILD, Kolkata,
West Bengal, India

PREFACE

Handwriting is often considered as an important aspect of daily life, yet its significance cannot be overstated. For many individuals, the ability to write legibly and efficiently is not only essential for academic and professional success but also for expressing oneself and engaging with the world. As Occupational Therapists, we understand the profound impact that handwriting difficulties can have on individual's confidence, independence, and overall well-being.

This book is born out of a shared passion for empowering individuals to overcome handwriting challenges and reach their full potential. Drawing from our collective experiences as Occupational Therapist, educators, and researchers, we have endeavored to create a comprehensive resource that addresses the multifaceted nature of handwriting intervention.

In the pages that follow, readers will find a wealth of information encompassing therapeutic techniques, activity ideas, and practical strategies tailored to diverse populations and settings. Whether working with children learning to form their first letters, adolescents striving to keep pace with academic demands, or adults relearning handwriting skills following injury or illness, this book offers guidance and support to every step of the way.

We firmly believe in the value of evidence-based practice, and as such, each recommendation presented in this book is grounded in current research and clinical expertise. However, we also recognize the importance of flexibility and creativity in Occupational Therapy intervention.

It is our hope that this book will serve as a trusted companion for Occupational Therapist navigating the complex terrain of handwriting intervention. Whether used as a reference for quick tips or as a comprehensive guide for developing structured intervention plans, we trust that readers will find valuable insights and practical solutions within these pages.

We extend our deepest gratitude to our colleagues, mentors, clients, and families who have supported us on this journey. Without their unwavering encouragement and inspiration, this book would not have been possible.

As we embark on this exploration of handwriting in Occupational Therapy, let us remain steadfast in our commitment to empowering individuals of all ages and abilities to communicate, create, and connect through the written word.

Happy Writing!
Prof. Raghuram P

ACKNOWLEDGEMENT

Writing this "Raghuram's Occupational Therapy- The Handwriting Revolution: Scribble to Script" has been a labor of love and dedication, and I owe my gratitude to numerous individuals and institutions who have supported me throughout this endeavor.

I extend my appreciation to **Sri Ramachandra Institute of Higher Education and Research** (DU) for their resources, facilities, and the opportunity that has been contributed to the content of this book.

I am grateful to our respected **Chancellor, Pro - Chancellor, Vice - Chancellor, Pro - Vice Chancellor, Registrar and Additional Registrar** for their valuable support.

I thank respected **Ms. Sumathi Eswaran**, Ex- Vice Principal, MCOT, for her blessings and support.

I thank **Dr. P. Sankar, Chief Librarian, SRIHER** for his valuable support. Extending my thanks to **Mr. L. Bhaskaran, Superintendent, Administration, SRIHER** for his continuous support.

I thank the **Office Bearers of All India Occupational Therapists' Association (AIOTA).** Special mention to **Prof. P. Ramachandran, Ex - Head, Department of Paediatrics, SRMC & RI,** Porur, Chennai for his continuous support and guidance.

I am profoundly thankful to my mentors and colleagues in the field of Occupational Therapy who have provided guidance, shared their expertise, and challenged me to strive for excellence.

My dedicated research team deserves special recognition for their tireless efforts in collecting and analyzing data, as well as for their contributions to the research that underpins this book. My family and friends have provided unwavering support, understanding, and encouragement during long hours of research and writing.

I want to acknowledge the pioneering researchers and Occupational Therapy professionals whose work has inspired me throughout my career.

This book is a testament to the collective efforts and collaboration of these remarkable individuals and institutions. I am truly humbled by your support and grateful for the opportunity to contribute to the field of Occupational Therapy.

With Warm Regards,
– Prof. Raghuram P

AUTHOR AND CONTRIBUTORS

Author:
Prof. Raghuram P,
Head, Sri Ramachandra Faculty of Occupational Therapy (SRFOT),
Sri Ramachandra Institute of Higher Education and Research (DU),
Porur, Chennai.

Co-Authors:
Dr. Jose Mary Sangeetha. X (OT),
Occupational Therapist,
Department of Physical Medicine Rehabilitation (PMR)
JIPMER (Govt. of. India),
Puducherry.

Dr. Loganathan S (OT),
Assistant Professor,
Sri Ramachandra Faculty of Occupational Therapy (SRFOT),
Sri Ramachandra Institute of Higher Education and Research (DU),
Porur, Chennai.

Dr. T. Sundaresan (OT),
Assistant Professor,
Sri Ramachandra Faculty of Occupational Therapy (SRFOT),
Sri Ramachandra Institute of Higher Education and Research (DU),
Porur, Chennai.

Contributors:

Ms. Aarthi. A,
(M.O.T - Pediatrics),
Sri Ramachandra Faculty of Occupational Therapy (SRFOT),
Sri Ramachandra Institute of Higher Education and Research (DU),
Porur, Chennai.

Ms. Deepika. P,
(M.O.T - Pediatrics),
Sri Ramachandra Faculty of Occupational Therapy (SRFOT),
Sri Ramachandra Institute of Higher Education and Research (DU),
Porur, Chennai.

Ms. Kaviya. D,
(M.O.T - Neurology),
Sri Ramachandra Faculty of Occupational Therapy (SRFOT),
Sri Ramachandra Institute of Higher Education and Research (DU),
Porur, Chennai.

Ms. Kiruthika. K,
(M.O.T - Neurology),
Sri Ramachandra Faculty of Occupational Therapy (SRFOT),
Sri Ramachandra Institute of Higher Education and Research (DU),
Porur, Chennai.

Ms. Mona. E,
(M.O.T - Pediatrics),
Sri Ramachandra faculty of Occupational Therapy (SRFOT),
Sri Ramachandra Institute of Higher Education and Research (DU),
Porur, Chennai.

Ms. Monisha. T,
(M.O.T - Pediatrics),
Sri Ramachandra Faculty of Occupational Therapy (SRFOT),
Sri Ramachandra Institute of Higher Education and Research (DU),
Porur, Chennai.

Mr. Privin Raj. P
(M.O.T - Pediatrics),
Sri Ramachandra Faculty of Occupational Therapy (SRFOT),
Sri Ramachandra Institute of Higher Education and Research (DU),
Porur, Chennai.

Ms. Sowmia. S
(M.O.T - Pediatrics),
Sri Ramachandra Faculty of Occupational Therapy (SRFOT),
Sri Ramachandra Institute of Higher Education and Research (DU),
Porur, Chennai.

Ms. Suganthi. R
(M.O.T – Pediatrics),
Sri Ramachandra Faculty of Occupational Therapy (SRFOT),
Sri Ramachandra Institute of Higher Education and Research (DU),
Porur, Chennai.

Ms. Sweatha. I
(M.O.T - Pediatrics),
Sri Ramachandra Faculty of Occupational Therapy (SRFOT),
Sri Ramachandra Institute of Higher Education and Research (DU),
Porur, Chennai.

Ms. Shanmugapriya. V
(M.O.T - Pediatrics),
Sri Ramachandra Faculty of Occupational Therapy (SRFOT),
Sri Ramachandra Institute of Higher Education and Research (DU),
Porur, Chennai.

Ms. Uvanthiga. E
(M.O.T - Pediatrics),
Sri Ramachandra Faculty of Occupational Therapy (SRFOT),
Sri Ramachandra Institute of Higher Education and Research (DU),
Porur, Chennai.

Mr. Yashwanth. S. P
(M.O.T - Hand and Musculoskeletal Rehabilitation),
Sri Ramachandra Faculty of Occupational Therapy (SRFOT),
Sri Ramachandra Institute of Higher Education and Research (DU),
Porur, Chennai.

INTRODUCTION

Handwriting can be defined as a codified system of a finite number of standard symbols that exist in a specific language. Handwriting is a fundamental skill that humans have developed and refined over centuries, playing a crucial role in communication, education, and personal expression.

It has a rich history that dates back thousands of years. Early humans used various tools such as sticks, reeds, and feathers dipped in ink or pigment to inscribe symbols on surfaces like clay tablets, papyrus, and parchment. As writing systems evolved, so did the techniques and styles of handwriting.

A person's handwriting can convey their personality, emotions, and even cultural background. Handwriting and drawing have been considered as learned motor tasks.

It involves the process of forming letters, figures, or other significant symbols, predominantly on paper. Writing and drawing can be used to record experiences or thoughts, as well as to communicate with others.

Handwriting is a complex motor skill that can be improved through practice, repetition, feedback, and reinforcement. Handwriting is more than a motor skill; it requires connecting the letter name with a letterform and recalling a clear visual picture of the letterform from memory, as well as being able to execute the motor pattern required to produce the form.

Play is an important way in which young children gain essential knowledge and skills. Play is an essential strategy for learning and teaching. Play helps children to develop their milestones for handwriting.

Occupational Therapists provide varied practice for students, as well as sharing their knowledge of fine motor, visual motor, visual perceptual, motor planning, bodily kinesthetics, and attentional delays that might have an impact on the activity demands of the skill of making letters and words on a page. The ability to take notes accurately, legibly, and swiftly during a lecture can result in an increased ability to review and retain academic information. The role of the Occupational Therapist includes evaluating the child's developmental milestone and functional performance of prewriting and handwriting skills, along with the task demands and environmental features.

SKILLED HANDWRITING:

For an individual to perform a skilled handwriting, there are three level of considerations:

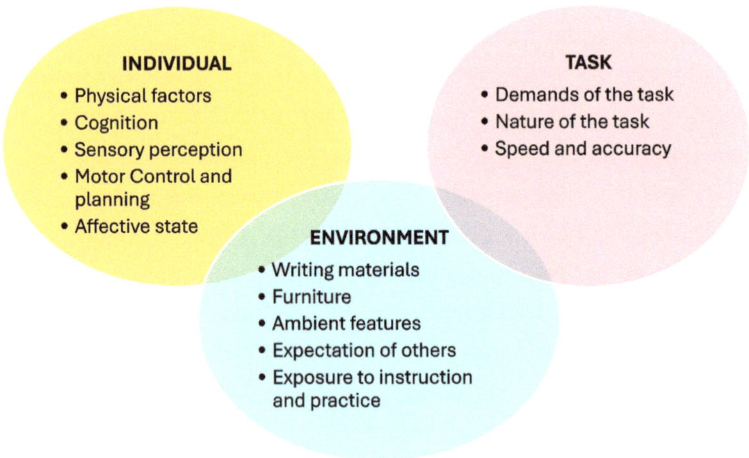

COMPONENTS OF HANDWRITING:

The components of handwriting can be broken down into categories: motor, visual perceptual, executive skill, and sensory.

SENSORY **MOTOR**

VISUAL PERCEPTUAL **EXECUTIVE SKILL**

HANDWRITING

MOTOR COMPONENTS:

- Range of motion
- Muscle strength
- Eye hand coordination
- Pencil control
- Fine motor skills
- Letter formation
- Letter size
- Speed
- Sitting posture

SENSORY COMPONENTS:

- Pencil pressure
- Body awareness
- Position in space (or proprioception)
- Self-regulation

VISUAL PERCEPTUAL COMPONENTS:

- Legibility
- Alignment
- Discrimination of letters
- Spatial awareness
- Figure ground perception

EXECUTIVE SKILL COMPONENTS:

- Working memory
- Impulse control
- Attention
- Organization
- Flexible thinking
- Planning and prioritization

SUMMARY:

Handwriting is a versatile and enduring form of communication and expression that continues to play an important role in academic activities and daily life routine.

PRE - REQUISITES SKILLS FOR HANDWRITING

The Pre-requisites skills for handwriting can be broken down into several categories: sensory, motor, visual perceptual and executive skills. Each of the building pieces contribute to handwriting issues when there is a delay in advancement or issues with building the basic aptitudes upon the other expertise components.

SENSORY PROCESSING SKILLS:

Many people do not realize how impactful an integrated sensory system can be on the development and refinement of handwriting.

- **Tactile:** The ability to discriminate the feel of the pencil in hands to know how to properly grasp it.
- **Proprioceptive:** The ability to have a good sense of body awareness to accurately judge how much pressure to push with the pencil and how hard or how soft to grasp the pencil.
- **Vestibular:** The ability to maintain the head in an upright position and proper body posture.
- **Visual:** The ability to accurately judge and plan the use of the lines writing on the paper, and be able to block out irrelevant visual stimuli in the environment that would distract and to notice the size and orientation of letters.

FINE MOTOR SKILLS:

Fine motor skill is the ability to precisely utilize the hand and fingers in a skilled activity. Good hand function is dependent on the balance between the extrinsic and intrinsic muscles of the hand.

- **Pencil Grasp:** Fine motor skills are necessary for establishing and maintaining an appropriate pencil grasp, such as the tripod grasp or quadruped grasp. A functional pencil grasp allows individuals to hold the writing utensil with control and precision, facilitating smooth and efficient handwriting.
- **Grip Strength and Pressure:** Fine motor skills include grip strength, which is necessary for maintaining a secure grasp on the writing tool while applying controlled pressure on the paper. Adequate grip strength ensures that individuals can write comfortably and legibly without experiencing hand fatigue or cramping.
- **Crossing the midline:** Crossing the midline is an important developmental milestone and motor skill that plays a significant role in handwriting. The midline refers to an imaginary line that divides the body into left and right halves. Crossing the midline involves using the hand or foot to move across the body's midline to perform tasks on the opposite side.

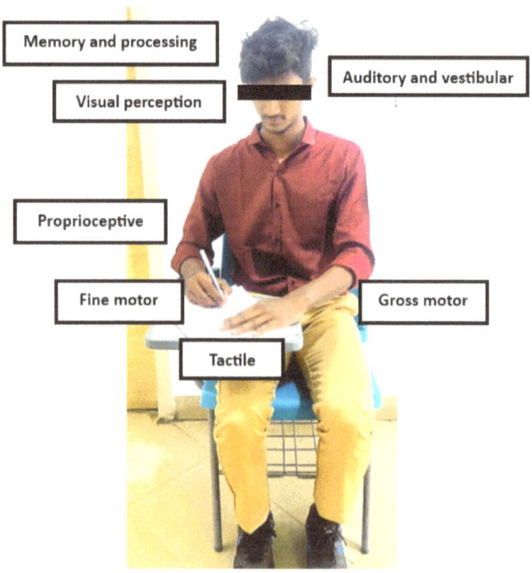

FINE MOTOR ELEMENTS: The fine motor skills can be further sub-categorized into a list:

BODY AWARENESS:

Body awareness is an essential part of handwriting, as it involves understanding and coordinating movements of the body, particularly the hands and arms, in relation to the writing task.

Here's how body awareness relates to handwriting:

- **Proximal Stability:** Proximal stability refers to stability around the core and proximal joints, such as the shoulder and elbow. Proximal stability is essential for controlling the movements of the arms and hands during handwriting, allowing for precise and coordinated movements without excessive tension or fatigue. By improving proximal stability, individuals can often improve their handwriting and overall fine motor skills. Proximal stability controls the distal mobility.
- **Postural Control**: Body awareness includes awareness of body posture and alignment, which are crucial for maintaining stability and support during handwriting. Individuals need to sit or stand in a stable position with proper alignment of the spine, shoulders, and arms to facilitate controlled movements of the hands and fingers during writing.
- **Core Stability**: Body awareness encompasses awareness of core stability, which refers to the strength and stability of the muscles in the abdomen, back, and pelvis. Core stability provides a solid foundation for upper body movements and helps to maintain proper posture and alignment during handwriting tasks.
- **Spatial Awareness:** Body awareness contributes to spatial awareness, which involves understanding the position, size, and spacing of letters and words. Spatial awareness help

individuals to maintain consistent letter size, spacing, and alignment, resulting in legible and organized handwriting. Spatial awareness in handwriting refers to the ability to accurately judge and control the placement and spacing of letters, words, and lines on a page. It involves understanding the relationship between individual letters, words, and the overall layout of written text. Strong spatial awareness skills are essential for producing legible and well-organized handwriting.

REFLEX INTEGRATION:

Reflex Integration in handwriting refers to the process of addressing and integrating primitive reflexes that may be persisting beyond the typical developmental stages and interfering with the fine motor control necessary for handwriting.

- **Asymmetric Tonic Neck Reflex (ATNR)**: This reflex occurs when the head is turned to one side, causing the limbs on that side to extend while the limbs on the opposite side flex. If the ATNR persists beyond infancy, it can interfere with bilateral coordination necessary for handwriting.
- **Symmetrical Tonic Neck Reflex (STNR)**: The STNR is triggered by changes in head position, causing extension of the arms and flexion of the legs when the head is extended, and flexion of the arms and extension of the legs when the head is flexed. Persistent STNR can disrupt eye-hand coordination and fine motor control needed for handwriting.
- **Palmar Reflex**: This reflex causes the fingers to curl inward in response to pressure on the palm of the hand. If the palmar reflex persists, it can result in applying more grip on writing tools, leading to difficulties with handwriting fluidity and control.
- **Grasp Reflex**: Like the palmar reflex, the grasp reflex causes the fingers to automatically close around objects placed in the

hand. Persistent grasp reflex can interfere with the ability to manipulate the writing tools effectively and maintain a proper pencil grip.

- **Moro Reflex**: Often referred to as the startle reflex, the moro reflex is triggered by sudden changes in sensory input, such as loud noises or sudden movements. If the moro reflex persists, it can cause involuntary jerk movements or tremors in the hands, impacting handwriting stability and legibility.

VISUAL PERCEPTION:

Visual perception plays a major role in handwriting as it involves the ability to interpret and make sense of visual information related to letters, words, and spatial relationships on a page.

The following is how visual perception relates to handwriting:

- **Letter Recognition:** Visual perception enables individuals to recognize and distinguish between different letters of the alphabet. While writing, the individuals must accurately perceive the shapes, sizes, and orientation of letters to reproduce it on the paper.
- **Visual Discrimination:** Visual discrimination refers to the ability to identify similarities and differences between the visual stimuli. In handwriting, visual discrimination allows the individuals to differentiate the patterns of alphabets **(e.g., "b" and "d")** and maintain consistency in letter formation.
- **Letter Formation:** Visual perception guides the process of letter formation by providing feedback on the sequence of strokes and spatial arrangement of lines and curves. Individuals use visual perception to monitor their writing and adjust letter shapes and proportions as needed.
- **Visual Memory:** Visual perception also involves visual memory, which is the ability to remember and recall visual information. Visual memory allows individuals to recognize

and reproduce familiar letter shapes and words from memory, facilitating fluent and spontaneous handwriting.

- **Visual - Motor Integration**: Visual perception is closely linked to visual-motor integration, which involves coordinating visual input with motor responses. In handwriting, visual perception guides hand movements to accurately reproduce letter shapes and strokes based on visual input from the written model.

EXECUTIVE FUNCTION SKILLS:

Executive function skills play an important role in handwriting, as it involves higher-level cognitive processes that governs planning, organization, and self-regulation.

Here's how executive function relates to handwriting:

- **Planning and Organization**: Executive function skills are essential for planning and organizing the writing process. Individuals must plan what they want to write, organize their thoughts into coherent sentences and paragraphs, and sequence their ideas logically. Poor executive function can lead to difficulties in initiating writing tasks, generating ideas, and structuring written work effectively.
- **Task Initiation and Time Management**: Executive function skills influence task initiation and time management during writing activities. Individuals with strong executive function can start writing tasks promptly and manage their time effectively to complete assignments within deadlines. Weak executive function may result in procrastination, difficulty getting started on writing tasks, and poor time management.
- **Attention and Concentration:** Attention and concentration are essential for sustaining focus and staying engaged in the writing process. Individuals must attend to the task, ignore distractions, and maintain concentration throughout the writing process. Effective attentional control allows the

individuals to allocate their cognitive resources efficiently, resulting in improved productivity and quality of writing.

- **Working Memory**: Working memory is a component of executive function that involves holding and manipulating information in the mind while performing cognitive tasks. Working memory is crucial for writing, as individuals must remember spelling rules, grammar conventions, and vocabulary words while composing the sentences and paragraphs. Poor working memory can lead to spelling errors, grammar mistakes, and difficulty with sentence structure.
- **Self-Monitoring and Error Correction**: Executive function skills support self-monitoring and error correction during writing. Individuals must monitor their writing for errors in spelling, grammar, punctuation, and content, and make appropriate revisions to improve clarity and coherence. Poor executive function may result in difficulties with self-monitoring, leading to errors and inconsistencies in written work.

SUMMARY:

This chapter explains the pre-requites skills required for handwriting and its importance. The prerequisites for handwriting encompass sensory processing skills, fine motor skills, body awareness, reflex integration, visual perception, and executive function Skills.

FINE MOTOR SKILLS

FINE MOTOR SKILLS:

Fine motor skills involve the coordination of small muscles in the hands and fingers with the eyes and brain. This development is essential for daily activities like writing, drawing, buttoning clothes, and using utensils. Children typically develop these skills through various milestones achieved in early childhood. The development of fine motor skills depends on the age-appropriate growth of physical abilities, such as core trunk control and shoulder strength, which provide a stable base for controlled arm and hand movements. Pre-writing and fine motor skills are crucial for preschoolers before they begin learning to write.

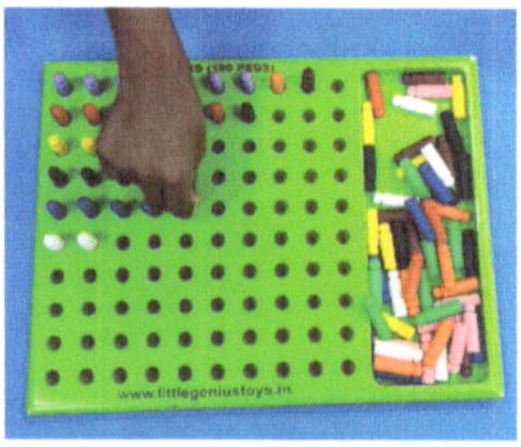

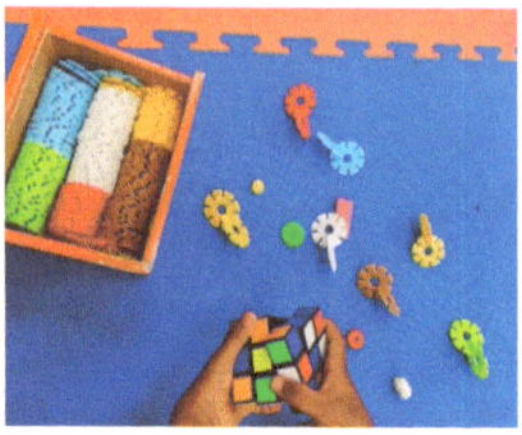

THE SIGNIFICANCE OF THE FINE MOTOR SKILLS IN CHILDHOOD DEVELOPMENT

- Fine motor skills enable children to perform basic self-care tasks independently, such as buttoning clothes, zipping zippers, tying shoelaces, brushing teeth, and feeding themselves with utensils.

- Fine motor skills are closely linked to academic success, especially in early childhood education. Activities like holding a pencil correctly, cutting with scissors, and coloring within the lines help to develop eye-hand coordination, spatial awareness, and the ability to control small movements.
- Proficient fine motor skills are critical for developing legible handwriting. Children with well-developed fine motor skills can control pencil pressure, form letters accurately, and write with fluency.

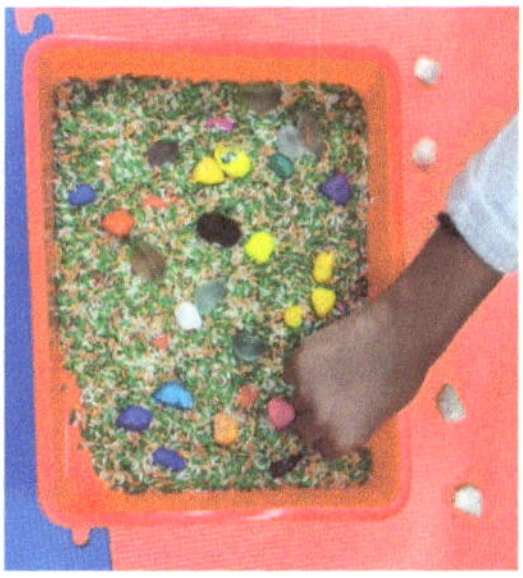

- Engaging in fine motor activities like arts and crafts, playing with small toys, or building with blocks fosters creativity, imagination, and self-expression. These activities also encourage social interaction, cooperation, and sharing when children engage in collaborative play, promoting positive social and emotional development.
- Fine motor skills are not only important in early childhood but also continue to be valuable throughout the life. Proficient fine motor abilities support the development of various life skills such as cooking, playing musical instruments, sports activities requiring eye-hand coordination, crafting, sewing, and woodworking. Overall, the development of fine motor skills in children is multi-faceted and influences various aspect of their physical, cognitive, social, emotional, and functional skills.

UNDERSTANDING DEVELOPMENTAL MILESTONES

Understanding developmental fine motor milestones helps the caregivers and educators to monitor a child's progress and provide appropriate support and interventions as needed. Following are a breakdown of key developmental fine motor milestones across different age:

- **Birth to 3 months**
  - Initial reflexes and discovering hands
- **3-6 months**
  - Grasping and reaching
- **6-9 months**
  - Improved hand control
- **9-12 months**
  - Pincer grasp and beginning scribbles
- **1-2 years**
  - Enhanced object manipulation, drawing, and beginning cutlery use
- **2-3 year**
  - Mastery of cutlery, improved drawing and stacking
- **3-4 years**
  - Enhanced drawing and cutting skills
- **4-5 years**
  - Writing and complex craft activities
- **5-6 years**
  - Precision in writing and complex crafts
- **Beyond 6 years**
  - Refinement and dexterity

AGE	DEVELOPMENTAL MILESTONES
Birth – 6 Months	• Reflexive grasp • Global ineffective reach for objects • Voluntary grasp • 2 handed palmar grasp • 1 handed palmar grasp • Controlled reach
7 – 12 Months	• Reaches, grasps, object in mouthing • Controlled release of objects • Static pincer grasp (thumb and index finger) • Pick things up with pincer grasp (thumb and index finger) • Transfer objects from one hand to another • Drops and picks up toys
1 - 2 Years	• Builds tower of three small blocks • Puts four rings on stick • Places five pegs in pegboard • Turns pages two or three of a book at a time • Scribbles • Turns knobs • Paints with whole arm movement, shifts hands, makes strokes • Self-feeds with minimal assistance • Able to use signing to communicate • Brings spoon to mouth • Holds and drinks from cup independently
2 - 3 Years	• Strings four large beads • Turns single pages of a book • Snips with scissors • Holds crayon with thumb and fingers (without fisting) • Uses one hand consistently in most activities • Imitates circular, vertical, and horizontal strokes • Paints with some wrist action, makes dots, lines, circular strokes • Rolls, squeezes, and pulls playdough • Eats without assistance

AGE	DEVELOPMENTAL MILESTONES
3 – 4 Years	• Builds tower of nine small blocks • Copies circle • Imitates cross • Manipulates clay material (rolls balls, makes snakes, cookies) • Uses non-dominant hand to assist and stabilize the use of objects • Snips paper using scissors
4 - 5 Years	• Cuts on line continuously • Copies cross • Copies square • Writes name • Writes numbers 1-5 • Copies letters • Hand dominance is well established • Dresses and undresses independently
5 – 6 Years	• Cuts out simple shapes • Copies triangle • Colors within the boundaries • Uses a 3 fingered grasp of pencil and uses fingers to generate movement • Can draw basic pictures
6 - 7 Years	• Forms most letters and numbers correctly • Writes consistently on the lines • Demonstrates controlled pencil movement • Established endurance for writing • Can build blocks independently • Ties shoelaces independently
7- 8 Years	• Maintains legibility of handwriting for entirety of a story

WHY TRACKING DEVELOPMENTAL MILESTONES ARE IMPORTANT?

Tracking fine motor developmental milestones is crucial for several important reasons, as outlined below:

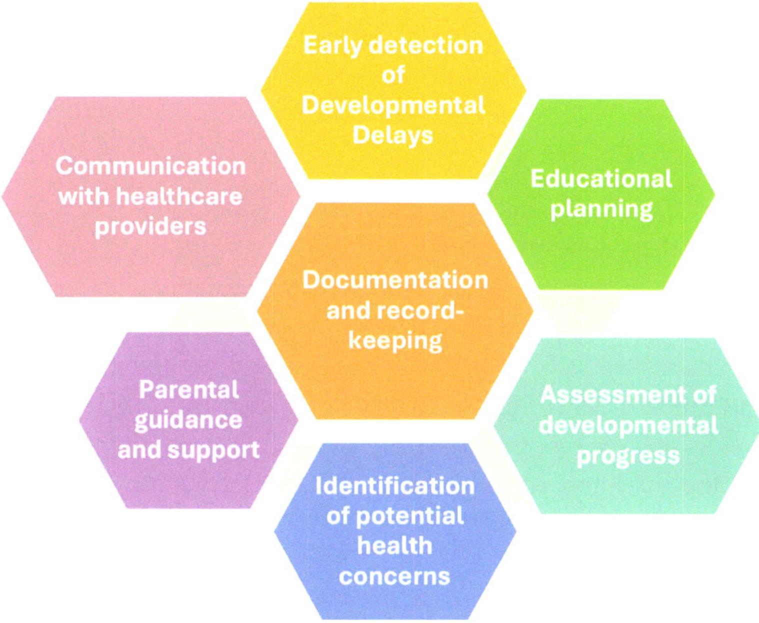

SUMMARY:

Fine motor skills start developing in infancy, and keep improving as kids get older. Developing and refining fine motor skills is essential for independence, academic success, and overall functional abilities throughout life. Practicing a variety of activities that target fine motor skill development can help individuals improve their dexterity, coordination, and control over hand and finger movements. By addressing and developing these fine motor skills and related abilities, individuals can improve their handwriting proficiency and overall fine motor control, leading to clearer and more legible written communication.

PRE - WRITING SKILLS

INTRODUCTION:

The essential fine motor abilities that children need to acquire before they develop writing are known as pre-writing skills. The child's grip strength, eye-hand coordination, and wrist movements can be facilitated with pre-writing skills. Children will then benefit from these when they learn to gradually hold and utilize a pencil or any other writing utensils to write, color, sketch, and express themselves in general. Pre - writing abilities are the lines and stroke patterns that children must learn and practice for writing development.

SKILLS THAT ARE REQUIRED FOR WRITING READINESS:

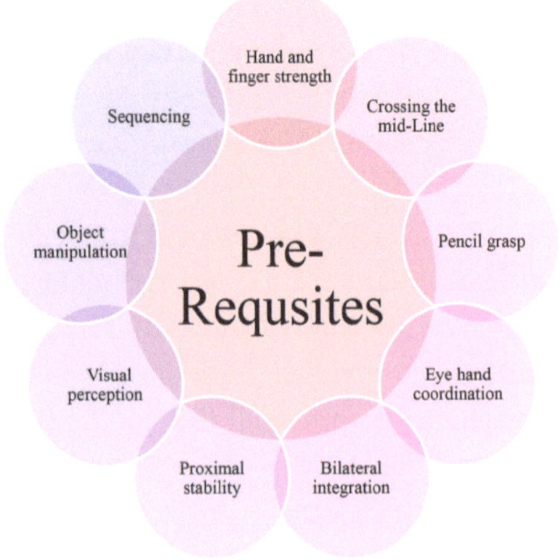

PRE-WRITING SKILLS MILESTONES:

Developmental milestones for prewriting skills vary among children but generally follow a progression from basic motor coordination to more refined control and planning.

Here are some typical developmental milestones for prewriting skills:

Age	Development
1-2 Years	• Randomly scribbles • Spontaneously scribbles in vertical / horizontal and/or circular motion • Imitates horizontal/vertical/circular direction • Grab a crayon with a palmar grasp and random scribbling
2-3 Years	• Imitates a horizontal line (—) • Imitates a vertical line (|) • Imitates a circle ◯
3-4 Years	• Copies a horizontal line (—) • Copies a vertical line (|) • Copies a circle ◯ • Imitates plus symbol (+) • Imitates / (right slanting line) and \ (left slanting line) • Imitates a square □
4-5 Years	• Copies a plus symbol (+) • Traces a line • Copies a square □ • Copies a / (right slanting line) and \ (left slanting line) • Imitates cross symbol (X) • Imitates triangle (Δ) • Grasp pencil in writing position • Colors within a picture with more than 0.25" deviation from the coloring line.
5-6 Years	• Copies cross symbol (X) • Copies triangle (Δ) • Recognizes between a big and small line or curve

These milestones provide a general framework for tracking the progression of pre-writing skills in children. However, it is important to remember that each child develops at their own pace, and individual differences should be considered when assessing writing readiness and skill acquisition. Additionally, providing ample opportunities for practice, exploration, and guidance can support children in reaching their full potential in pre-writing skills development.

IF A CHILD HAS DIFFICULTIES WITH WRITING READINESS THEY MIGHT:

- Have an awkward pencil grasp.
- Find it difficult to hold a pencil steadily while writing, coloring, or sketching.
- Exhibit a propensity to manipulate objects with their entire hand as opposed to only a few fingers.
- Have poor endurance for pencil-based activities.
- Write with sloppy or sluggish handwriting.
- Find it challenging to color inside the lines.
- When doing pencil-based tasks, apply the incorrect amount of pressure on the pencil (either too light or too heavy and often breaks the pencil).
- Lack of strength in upper limbs.
- Find it difficult to coordinate both hands when performing a task.
- Have poor eye – hand coordination.
- Possess strong verbal communication skills, but find it challenging to convey them in writing, drawing, or coloring.
- **Behavior**: The child may feel for using a pencil and other fine motor skills.
- **Avoidance:** The preference to have others guide them for the completion of fine motor activities rather than accomplishing them by themselves (e.g., "daddy, draw me a house" or "build me a rocket").
- **Self-esteem**: When individuals contrast their work with that of their colleagues.
- **Academic performance**: The child struggles harder and take longer time to finish these assignments, which slows down

the acquisition of new abilities (such as learning how to write their name or sketch a person).

STRATEGIES TO IMPROVE WRITING READINESS (PRE-WRITING) SKILLS?

- **Hand dominance**: Identify and support the dominant hand when performing precise tasks.
- **Experience**: Promote engagement in gripping and manipulating small objects tasks, like puzzles, drawing, opening containers, threading, and other similar activities.
- **Poking and pointing activities**: Play games that require to use of only one or two fingers at a time like drill finger motions.
- **Reinforce** and support the child in using their fine motor skills, especially if they persevere through challenging tasks.

➢ Drawing fun pictures or playing games of their choosing is a great way to build their pencil skills without tension.

- **Dexterity and Grip strength:**
  (e.g., utilizing tweezers, play dough, pegs, paper, and scrunching).

➢ Using different-sized laces for threading and lacing

➢ Teabag squeezers or tongs for picking up items.

➢ Routine tasks involving fingers, such as jar and container opening

➢ Scissor projects, which could entail cutting out geometric shapes and pasting them together to create images of houses, trains, or robots

- **Craft:** Create something out of paper, wool, egg cartons, and old boxes.
- **Sensory play** that promotes the development of tactile awareness, including finger painting and rice play.
- **Playdough activities:** These can include rolling with a rolling pin or hands, finding hidden things in the playdough, or just making things creatively.

- ➢ Practice forming strokes or shapes in sand or foam in a playful manner
- ➢ Practice writing pre-printing shapes, letters, sight words, and spellings.
- **Eye – hand coordination**:
- ➢ Practice tasks requiring this ability, such as tossing and catching, as well as crossing the midline, such as reaching across the body to pick something up.
- ➢ Writing or drawing on a vertical surface.
- **Pre-writing forms:** Get comfortable sketching the following: l, —, O, +, /, square, \, X, and Δ.

SUMMARY:

Pre-writing skills are essential to fine motor abilities that children need before they start writing. These skills include grip strength, eye-hand coordination, and wrist movements. Developmental milestones for pre-writing skills progress from basic motor coordination to more refined control and planning, involving tasks like imitating lines and shapes. Difficulties with writing readiness might manifest as awkward pencil grasp, poor endurance, or sloppy handwriting. Strategies to improve pre-writing skills include promoting hand dominance, engaging in gripping activities, playing finger games, reinforcing fine motor skills through drawing, and enhancing dexterity and grip strength through various activities like sensory play and crafting.

WRITING SKILL DEVELOPMENT

INTRODUCTION:

Writing skill development is an important part of a child's educational journey since it involves a variety of cognitive, physical, and linguistic abilities. From scribbling the first marks on paper to composing coherent essays in high school, the evolution of writing proficiency reflects the maturing of several domains of development. Understanding age-appropriate milestones and supporting children in developing their writing skills are critical for effective communication and academic performance.

STAGES OF WRITING DEVELOPMENT:

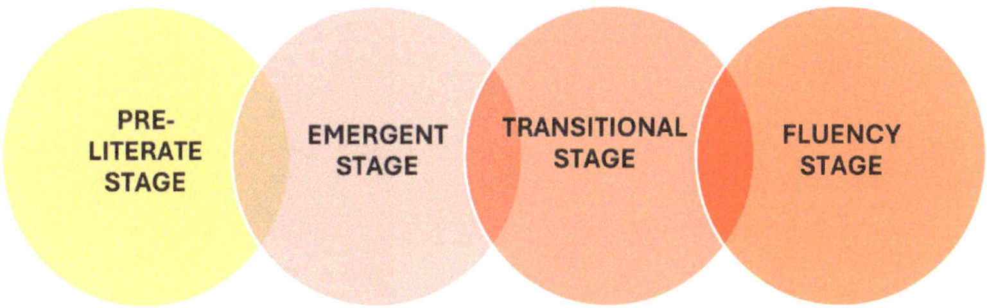

PRE- LITERATE STAGE (0-2 YEARS)	
S.NO	**STAGE DESCRIPTION**
1	**Scribble stage** - Making large circular strokes and random marks anywhere on the page that don't look like writing or convey any message.
2	**Symbolic stage** - Creating pictures or random marks anywhere on the page with the intention of conveying a message.
3	**Directional Scribble** - Producing linear scribbles from left to right, intended to resemble writing that conveys a meaningful message or idea.
4	**Symbolic/Mock letters** - Formations that look similar to letters but aren't intentionally created as such, often mixed with numbers and lacking proper spacing.

EMERGENT STAGE (2-4 YEARS)	
S.NO	**STAGE DESCRIPTION**
1	**String of Letters** - Long sequences of randomly ordered letters, typically moving left to right, often using letters from one's name, usually in capital letters, and sometimes repeating letters in different forms.
2	**Group of Letters** - Clusters of letters separated by spaces to mimic the appearance of words.
3	**Labeling Pictures** - Using the initial sound of a word to match it with the corresponding letter to label a picture.
4	**Environmental Print** - Replicates letters or words from surroundings or classroom print, often includes reversals, and utilizes various resources to aid writing.

TRANSITIONAL STAGE (4-7 YEARS)	
S.NO	**STAGE DESCRIPTION**
1	**Letter/Word Representation** - Utilizes the initial sound of a word to represent the whole word, employing letter-sound associations.
2	**First/Last Letter Representation** - Word depicted by the sounds of its initial and final letters.
3	**Medial Letter Sounds** - Words spelled phonetically employing beginning, middle, and end sounds, including attempts at representing medial vowels. Incorporates familiar and more conventionally spelled words, with one letter typically representing each syllable. Efforts to include word spacing enhance readability.

FLUENT STAGE (8-10 YEARS)	
S.NO	**STAGE DESCRIPTION**
1	**Initial Phrase Writing** - Applying the aforementioned skills to compose phrases that convey a message corresponding to their illustration.
2	**Sentence Composition** - Organizing words into coherent sentences, potentially comprising multiple sentences. Writing is legible, may incorporate punctuation, correctly spelled familiar words, and maintains a focused topic. Utilizes beginning, middle, and end structure with added detail.
3	**Six Traits of Writing** - Students employ six key aspects of writing: conventions, organization, voice, ideas, word choice, and sentence fluency.

WRITING DEVELOPMENT AND COPING STRATEGIES:

1. Preliterate Stage (0 - 2 years):

- Children begin to make scribbles and marks that resemble writing.
- They experiment with holding writing tools and understanding that writing carries meaning.
- Letter-like forms may start to emerge, although not necessarily representing actual letters.

Strategies:

- A great way to encourage the child as a writer – even in this early stage – is to say, "Tell me what you wrote."
- Children enjoy telling stories, and it will make them enjoy learning about the frequently intricate and imaginative ideas that are behind those simple scribbles.
- Ensure that the child has easy access to paper, crayons, and markers so they may begin writing whenever inspiration strikes. Pens and pencils are acceptable as well, although young children frequently find it easier to grasp thicker tools for writing.

- Another way that may support the child is by sending her notes. A note return can be motivated with a simple one that says, "I love you!" left on the breakfast table.

2. Emergent Stage (2 - 4 years):

- Children start forming recognizable letters, usually beginning with uppercase letters.
- They develop basic phonemic awareness, associating sounds with letters.
- Writing consists of simple words and short, phonetically-spelled sentences.

Strategies:

- The child will discover that letters form words when you teach him/her to write his/her name. Additionally, it promotes the transition from sloppy writing to the use of letters as symbols. That can then teach him/her to write words like "Mom," "Dad," and the names of other family members once he/she has mastered that.
- Making signs for role-playing games, like a STOP sign for when you are playing vehicles, is another interesting concept.
- Reading will be essential at this stage as well. Making time every day to read a book to the child is an effective way to foster reading skills. Reading aloud to a child not only nurtures a love of reading but also awakens his inner storyteller. The child will begin to conceive of his/her own imaginative stories. The concepts that words are composed of letters and have meanings are also reinforced by reading aloud. For numerous children, this practice not only leads to reading but also to writing. For instance, a child will begin to know the word "bug" after seeing it multiple times in a story. When he realises that, he/she can proceed to write those three letters so he/she can share his/her own bug story.

3. Transitional Stage (4 - 7 years) :

- Children refine letter formation and begin using lowercase letters consistently.
- They expand their vocabulary and sentence structure, incorporating more complex words and phrases.
- Writing becomes more legible, and children start to apply basic punctuation and capitalization rules.

Strategies:

Incorporate pretend play into the writing to motivate as a transitional writer. With his/her toys, assist child in writing a menu for a tea party or a prescription for you when you're pretending to be a doctor. Save these tiny treasures. Years from now, you'll both love trying to figure out how the invented spelling worked out.

4. Fluent Writing Stage (8 - 10 years):

- Children write with increasing fluency and sophistication, demonstrating a grasp of grammar and syntax.
- They can organise their thoughts into paragraphs and essays, using a variety of sentence structures.
- Writing shows evidence of revision and editing for clarity and coherence.

Strategies:

Encourage the child to write to communicate with others. Try sending brief notes to loved ones, friends, and each other. Writing shared stories is another entertaining method to turn writing into a group activity.

HANDWRITING DEVELOPMENTAL MILESTONES

AGE	DEVELOPMENTAL MILESTONES
1 - 2 years	• Palmar supinate grasp emerges. • Engages in haphazard scribbling. • Shows spontaneous scribbling in vertical, horizontal, or circular directions. • Imitates scribbling in horizontal, vertical, or circular patterns
2 – 3 years	• Digital pronate grasp emerges. • Imitates drawing a horizontal and vertical line. • Attempts to replicate a circle shape.
3 – 4 years	• Initial development of static tripod grasp. • Successfully cuts a piece of paper in half. • Reproduces a horizontal and a vertical line. • Replicates a circle shape. • Attempts to mimic the symbols "+", "/", "". • Tries to imitate a square shape
4 - 5 years	• Static tripod or quadruped grasp further develops. • Able to cut out large shapes such as circles and squares with scissors. • Capable of drawing a person with a minimum of three distinct body parts. • Successfully reproduces the symbols "+", "/". • Demonstrates the ability to trace lines. • Copies a square shape accurately. • Imitates the shapes of an "X" and a triangle "Δ".
5 - 6 years	• Both dynamic tripod and quadruped grasps are in development. • Hand dominance (either right or left-handed) continues to evolve and solidify. • Capable of drawing a person with six or more body parts. • Able to color within lines neatly. • Begins to write numerals 1- 5. • Can write their name using either uppercase or lowercase letters. • Recognizes the distinction between big and small lines or curves.
6 - 7 years	• Successfully forms most letters and numbers accurately. • Maintains consistent alignment with writing on the lines. • Exhibits controlled movements with the pencil. • Demonstrates good endurance when writing.
7 - 8 years	• Sustains legible handwriting consistently throughout the story.

GRASP PATTERN:

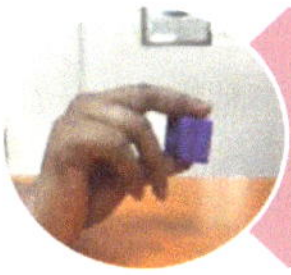

RADIAL DIGITAL GRASP
6 Months

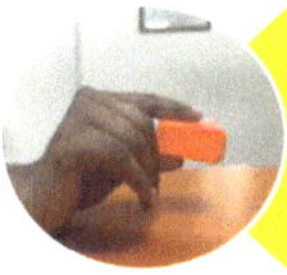

INFERIOR PINCER GRASP
9 Months

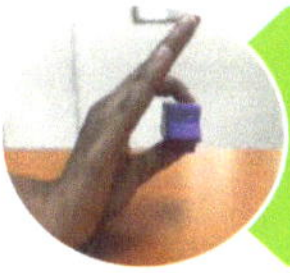

REFINED PINCER GRASP
12 Months

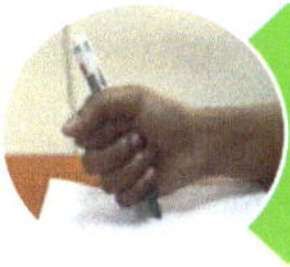

PALMAR SUPINATE GRASP
12 Months

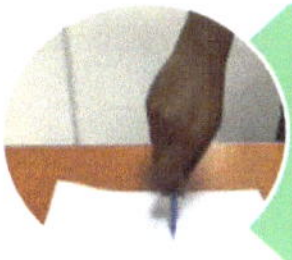

DIGITAL PRONATE GRASP
2 Years

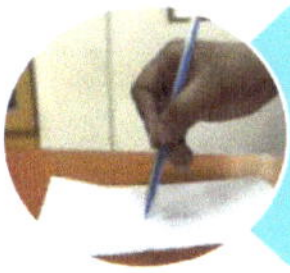

STATIC TRIPOD GRASP
3.5 Years

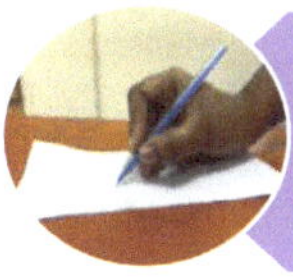

DYNAMIC TRIPOD GRASP
4.5 Years

FOUNDATION SKILLS FOR HANDWRITING:

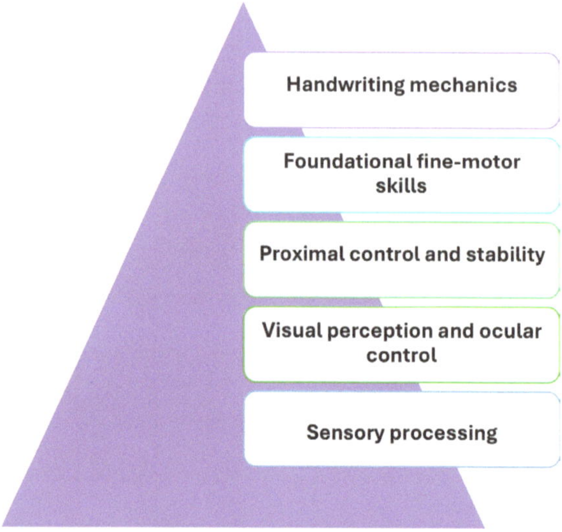

- **Sensory processing** - The process by which the body gathers, arranges, deciphers, and reacts to sensory input from our surroundings is known as sensory processing.
- **Visual perception and ocular control** - The way how the child his/her eyes and how the brain processes what they see.
- **Proximal control and stability** - Related to posture, core stability, and control.
- **Foundational fine motor skills** - Includes the hand musculature, as well as strength and dexterity.
- **Handwriting mechanics** – Placing the pencil on the paper, the actual writing part of handwriting.

Summary:

Writing skill development encompasses cognitive, physical, and linguistic abilities, evolving from scribbling to composing essays. Understanding age-appropriate milestones and supporting children are crucial for effective communication and academic performance.

4 P'S MANAGEMENT

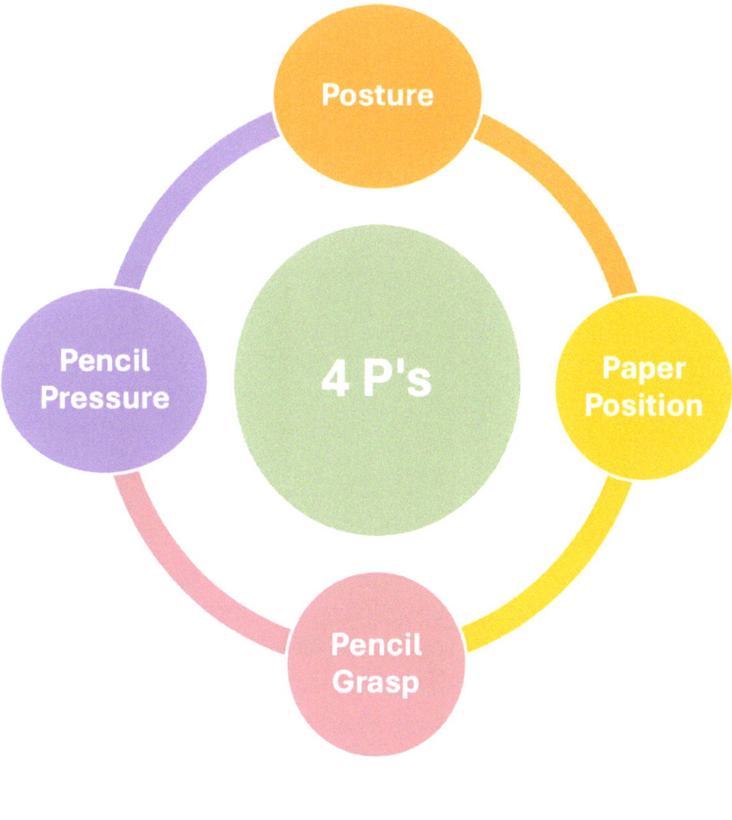

PENCIL GRASP: The development of a mature pencil grasp is explained as a sequence from primitive pencil grasp and transitional pencil grasp.

PRIMITIVE PENCIL GRASP

Writing tool stabilized in plam of hand.

Holding the writing tool with whole hand or extended fingers, forearm pronated and using the shoulder to move the pencil.

TRANSITIONAL PENCIL GRASP

Writing tool stabilized between thumb and fingers.

Writing tool held against index finger with thumb crossed over toward index finger

MATURE PENCIL GRASP

The pencil is stabilized by the distal phalanges of the thumb, index, middle and ring finger, the wrist is extended.

MATURE PENCIL GRASP PATTERNS

Here are four main and acceptable types of mature pencil grasp. These are the most used mature pencil grasp among various individuals.

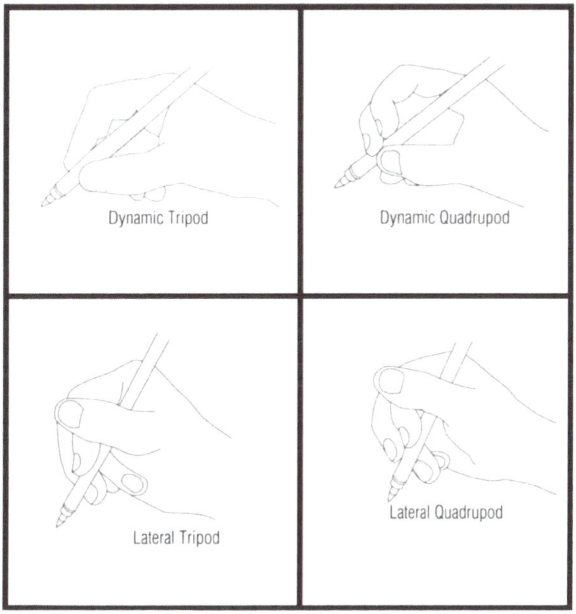

PENCIL PRESSURE:

- It is the amount of pressure applied on the writing tool.
- The child holds the pencil with a comfortable amount of pressure. The pencil should not be held with a strained force or a floppy grip.
- The pencil pressure should remain the same throughout the writing task.

PAPER POSITION:

- Paper should be slanted on the desktop so that it is parallel to the forearm of the writing hand when the child's forearms are resting on the desk with hands clasped.

- Right-handed individuals may slant the top of their paper approximately 25° to 30° to the left with the paper placed just right of the body's midline.
- Left-handed individuals - a slant of 30° to 35° to the right and paper placement to the left of midline are needed.

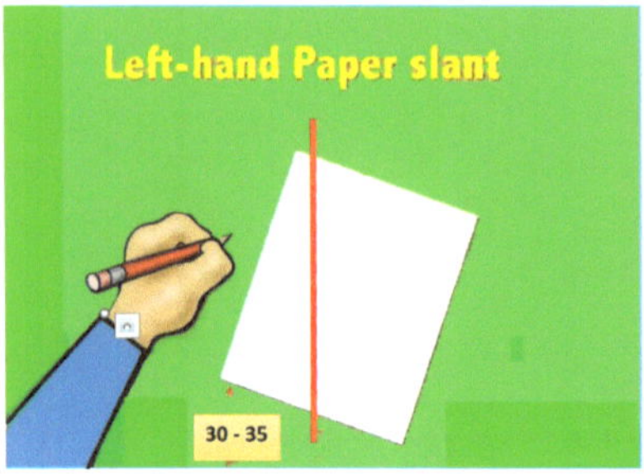

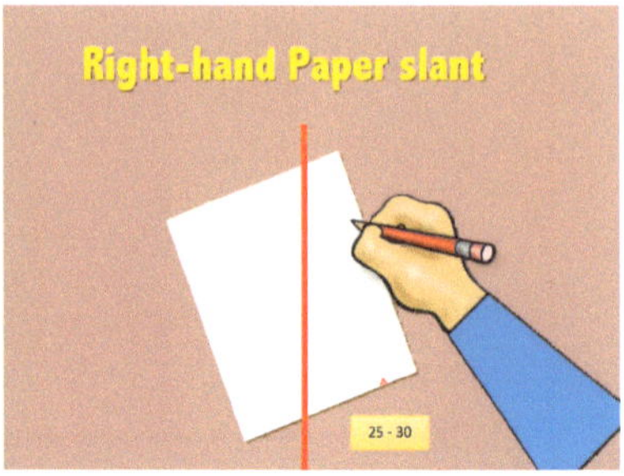

POSTURE:

- **Correct sitting posture for handwriting:** Knees and Hips flexed at 90° and feet flat on the floor. The writing surface is 2 inches above the student's bent elbow. The top of the chair should be slightly below the student's shoulder blade.
- Maintenance of an optimal posture while writing plays significant role in prevention of musculoskeletal discomfort.

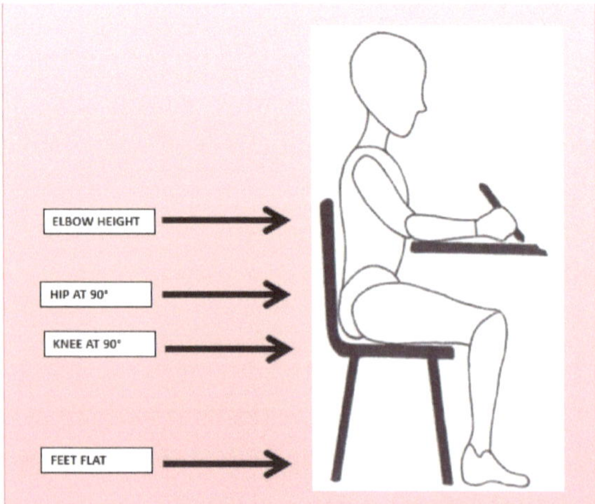

LETTER FORMATION, ALIGNMENT AND SPACING

LETTER FORMATION:

Letter formation refers to the process of creating individual letters using a series of strokes in a consistent and recognizable manner.

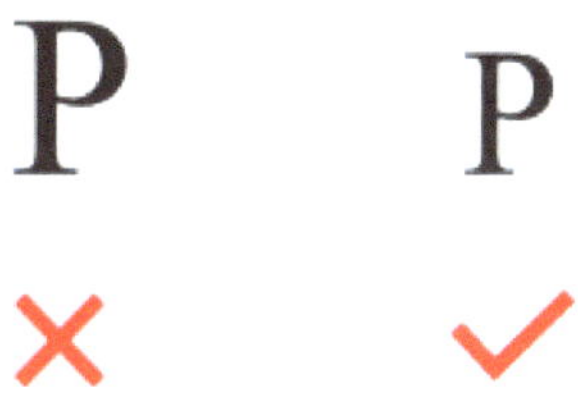

LETTER FORMATION INVOLVES 5 FEATURES:

- Improper letter forms,
- Poor leading in and out of letters
- Incomplete closure of letters
- Incorrect ascenders and descenders
- Inadequate rounding of letters

ERRORS IN LETTER FORMATION:

- **Letter stroke direction:** This refers to the direction in which strokes are made when forming letters, such as clockwise instead of anti-clockwise for letters like 'a' or 'o'. These errors are often noticed when reviewing the process of writing.

- **Starting place:** Some letters like 'r', 'n', or 'i' should begin at a specific point, typically in the middle of the lines rather than at the baseline.
- **Missing strokes:** Occur when essential strokes in letters, like the cross stroke in 't' and 'f', are omitted. Also, letters like 'r', 'n', or 'u' may be formed with only one stroke instead of the required two.
- **Added strokes:** This happens when extra strokes are added, often overwriting strokes that were already formed correctly.
- **Letter reversals:** Instances where letters are written in reverse, for example, 'b' appearing as 'd'.
- **Broad error categories:** These encompass various types of errors in letter formation, including spatial, cross midline, directionality, integration/close, integration/open, and distortions.

PRACTICE OF LETTER FORMATION (Desk work; one letter at a time)

- Repeat each letter with a rhythmic script as it is presented.
- Trace each letter and copy each letter from a visual model into a box on paper that has clear visual boundaries.
- Erase lines of letter in same sequence it was formed, with small sponge. Breaking down letters into individual strokes and practicing each stroke separately before combing them to form the compete letter can help learners focus on mastering each component.

SPACING:

- Spacing includes the dispersion of letters within words and words within sentences along with text organization on the entire sheet of paper. Effective spacing is crucial for legibility, readability, and overall aesthetic appeal of written text.

- **Optimal word spacing:** The recommended space between words is typically equivalent to the size of one lowercase letter.
- **Blank Space Consideration:** It's valuable to discuss the empty space between lines and across the entire page as well. Specify how the work is organized to make it easier to view and read through applying these gaps and spaces.

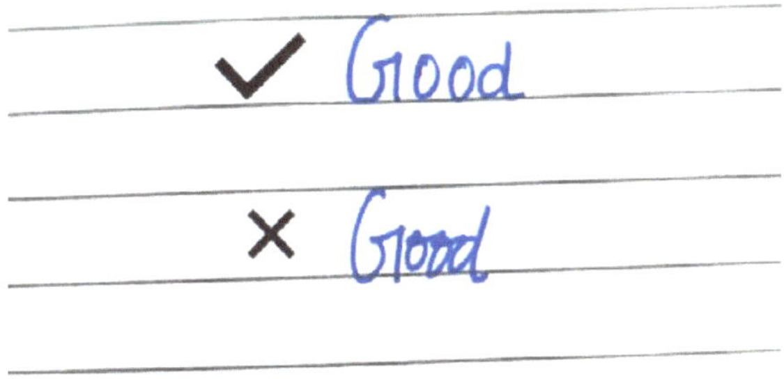

SPACING IN HANDWRITING INVOLVES SEVERAL ELEMENTS:

- **Letter spacing:** This refers to the distance between individual letters within a word. Proper letter spacing ensures that each letter is distinct and does not blend into adjacent letters, aiding in recognition and comprehension.
- **Word spacing:** Word spacing involves the consistent and appropriate distance between words within a sentence or paragraph. Adequate word spacing facilitates fluent reading by providing clear delineation between words and preventing them from running together.
- **Line spacing:** Line spacing, also known as line height or leading, refers to the vertical distance between lines of text. Proper line spacing ensures adequate separation between lines, preventing overcrowding and improving readability.
- **Margins:** Margins are the blank spaces surrounding the written text on a page. Adequate margins provide framing

for the text and allow for annotations or corrections without interfering with the readability of the main content.

EFFECTIVE SPACING IN HANDWRITING IS INFLUENCED BY VARIOUS FACTORS INCLUDING:

- **Motor control:** The ability to control hand movements plays a significant role in achieving consistent spacing. Individuals with fine motor difficulties may struggle to maintain uniform spacing due to challenges in controlling the movement of their writing instrument.
- **Visual perception:** Accurate spacing relies on visual perception to judge distances and proportions between letters, words, and lines. Difficulties in visual perception can lead to irregular spacing or overcrowding of text.
- **Spatial awareness:** Spatial awareness refers to the ability to understand and navigate the physical space around oneself. Strong spatial awareness enables individuals to accurately gauge distances and proportions, contributing to effective spacing in handwriting.

ALIGNMENT:

Alignment or baseline orientation refers to the placement of text on and within the writing guidelines. Handwriting alignment encompasses both horizontal (left-to-right) and vertical (top-to-bottom) positioning of text on the page. Proper alignment ensures that letters and words are evenly spaced and neatly organized, enhancing readability and visual appeal. However, challenges with alignment can lead to illegible or messy handwriting, affecting communication and academic performance.

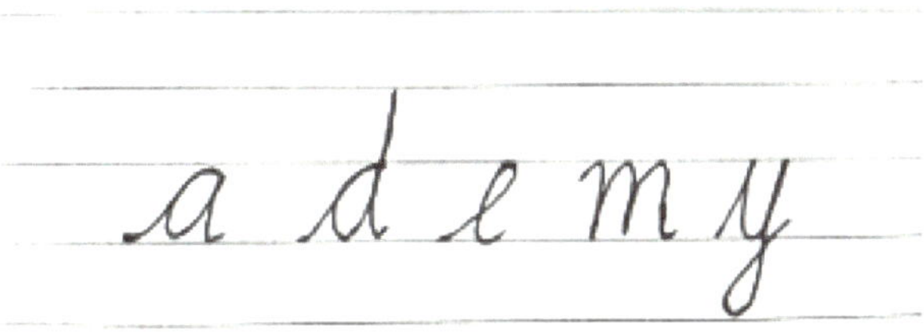

COMMON CHALLENGES WITH ALIGNMENT:

- **Horizontal alignment:** Difficulty maintaining a consistent left-to-right progression across the page, resulting in uneven spacing between words or sentences.
- **Vertical alignment:** Trouble keeping letters and words aligned along the baseline, leading to text that appears slanted or unevenly distributed vertically.
- **Spacing:** Inconsistent spacing between letters, words, or lines can disrupt alignment and overall legibility.
- **Letter formation:** Variability in the size and shape of individual letters can affect alignment, particularly when letters are not properly aligned vertically.

MANAGEMENT STRATEGIES:

Training the alignment component in handwriting involves a combination of targeted exercises, practice activities, and environmental modifications to improve both horizontal and vertical alignment. Here are some strategies for training alignment in handwriting:

- **Visual Cueing:** Use visual cues such as colored lines or dots to indicate where each letter should start and end, helping individuals align their writing along a baseline.
- **Modelling and Demonstration:** Demonstrate proper alignment by modelling handwriting on a whiteboard or large paper. Encourage individuals to observe and replicate the alignment of letters and words.

- **Handwriting warm-up activities**: Begin sessions with warm-up activities like tracing lines or shapes to promote eye–hand coordination and spatial awareness, laying the foundation for better alignment in handwriting.
- **Visual motor integration activities:** Engage in activities that integrate visual and motor skills, such as drawing shapes within designated boundaries or copying patterns with specific alignment requirements.
- **Vertical alignment exercises:** Practice writing on lined paper or graph paper to help individuals align letters and words vertically along the baseline. Encourage attention to the height and placement of letters relative to the lines.
- **Consistency drills:** Develop drills focused on consistency in letter size, spacing, and alignment. Encourage individuals to pay attention to the visual appearance of their writing and adjust as needed.

SUMMARY:

Letter formation involves creating letters in a consistent and recognizable manner, without errors including incorrect stroke direction, starting place, missing, or added strokes, and reversals. Practice methods include rhythmic repetition and tracing. Spacing in handwriting involves letter, word, and line spacing, crucial for readability and aesthetics. Effective spacing relies on motor control, visual perception, and spatial awareness. Alignment refers to horizontal and vertical positioning of text, with challenges including uneven spacing and slanted text. Management strategies for alignment training include visual cueing, modelling, warm-up activities, visual-motor integration, and consistency drills.

LEGIBILITY

WHAT IS LEGIBILITY?

Legibility refers to the characteristic of being clear and easy to read or understand. In the context of handwriting, legibility specifically refers to the readability of handwritten text, with the key concern being whether what the child wrote can be read by the child, parent, or a teacher.

FACTORS TO BE CONSIDERED FOR LEGIBLE HANDWRITING:

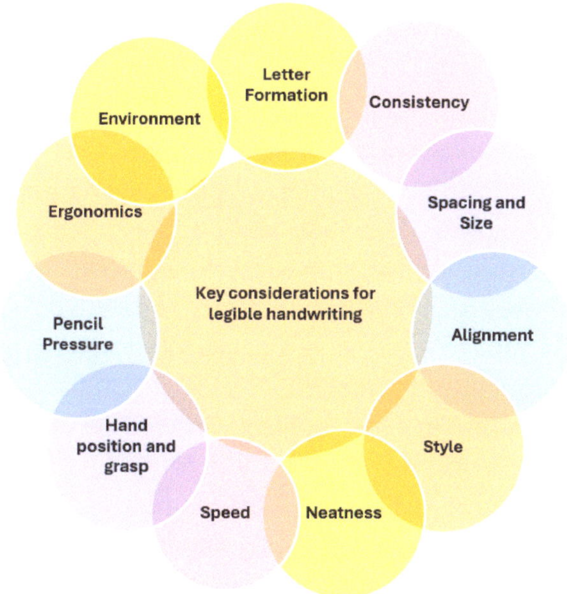

- **Letter formation**: Pay attention to the proper formation of each letter. Ensure that letters are recognizable and distinguishable from one another.
- **Consistency:** Maintain a consistent letter size, shape, and spacing throughout your written work. This uniformity improves comprehension as well as reading.
- **Spacing:** It includes the dispersion of letters within words and words within sentence.
- **Size:** It refers to the letter relative to the writing guidelines and to the other letters.
- **Alignment:** It refers to the positioning of text within and along the writing guidelines.
- **Style:** While everyone has a unique handwriting style, it is essential to ensure that your writing is clear and easily understandable by others.
- **Neatness:** Handwriting that is neat and tidy is often easier to read than messy or sloppy writing.
- **Speed:** A child's rate of writing, or the number of letters written per minute, and its readability are the two cornerstones of functional handwriting. Writing speed typically decreases when the amount of written work or the complex nature of the writing activity increase. Similarly, writing speed increases with age, familiar word production and practice.
- **Hand position and grip**: Hand position and grip refer to the way an individual holds and positions their hand while writing, which directly influences the legibility.
- **Pencil pressure**: Pencil pressure or the force exerted on the writing surface while using a pencil has a significant impact on the legibility of handwriting.
- **Ergonomics**: In the context of legible handwriting, ergonomics involves creating a writing environment and adopting writing techniques that promote comfort, efficiency, and optimal physical alignment, thus enhancing the legibility of handwriting.

- **Environment**: The environment for legible handwriting refers to the physical surroundings and conditions in which writing takes place, which can significantly impact the quality and clarity of handwriting.

WHEN IT IS LEGIBLE?

- It is easily and quickly recognized at first glance.
- Each letter should be clearly distinguishable from others.
- Consistent size and spacing.
- Correct use of punctuation and capitalization.
- Text is well-aligned on the baseline; letters are uniformly slanted.
- Proper spacing prevents words and sentences from looking cramped or crowded out.

WHEN IT IS ILLEGIBLE?

- It is not easily and quickly recognized out of context at first glance.
- It is poorly formed, distorted and reversed.
- Numerals/letters are joined, share the same part, or overlap to form individual numbers.
- It is mistaken with another letter or numeral.
- It is confused for a group of letters or numerals.
- The entire numeral is either missing or misplaced in sequence.

AGE-APPROPRIATE LEGIBILITY DEVELOPMENT:

Early scribbling (Age 2-3):

- Legibility is minimal as children primarily engage in random scribbling motions.
- These scribbles bear little resemblance to recognizable letters or symbols.

Emergent writing (Age 3-4):

- Legibility begins to emerge as children experiment with forming basic shapes and lines that resemble letters.
- Writing may be irregular and inconsistent, but some letters or symbols may be recognizable.

Letter formation (Age 4-5):

- Legibility improves as children concentrate on forming individual letters with more intention and control.
- Letters become more recognizable and show signs of proper orientation and directionality.

Basic writing skills (Age 5-6):

- Legibility continues to improve as children refine their ability to form letters consistently and accurately.
- Letters are more consistent in size and shape, with better spacing and alignment.

Transition to print (Age 6-7):

- Legibility further improves as children transition to manuscript handwriting.
- Letters are formed with increased accuracy and clarity, with attention to proper letter formation and spacing.

Cursive writing (Age 8-9):

- Legibility may initially decrease during the transition to cursive writing as children adapt to new letter formations and connections.
- Legibility improves with practice as children develop fluency and consistency in cursive handwriting.

Refinement and fluency (Age 10-12):

- Handwriting reaches a higher level of legibility as children refine their skills and become more fluent in writing.
- Letters are formed with greater speed and efficiency while maintaining clarity and precision.

Mature handwriting (Age 13+):

- Legibility peaks as individuals achieve maturity in their handwriting skills.

- Handwriting becomes clear, consistent, and easily readable, reflecting a high level of proficiency and refinement.

ILLEGIBLE PARAGRAPH:

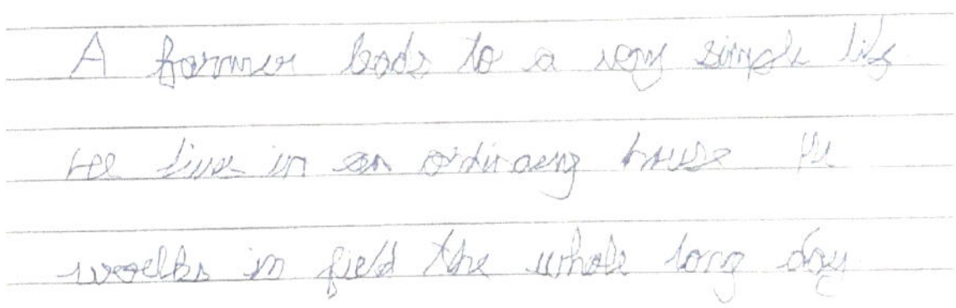

LEGIBLE PARAGRAPH:

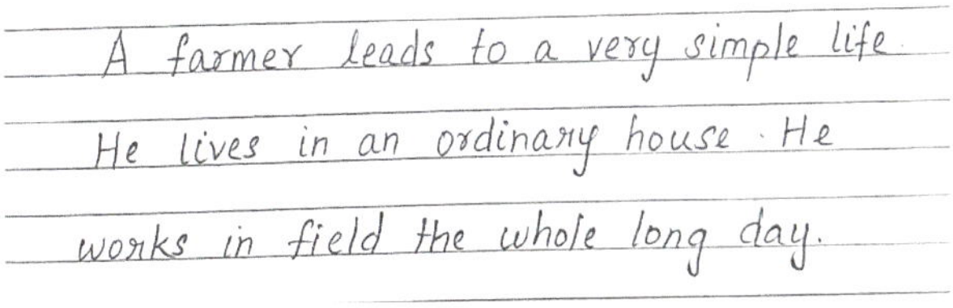

SUMMARY:

Handwriting legibility is an important ability that impacts communication, academic performance, and professional presentation. Achieving clear and readable handwriting ensures that written text is easily understood, preventing miscommunication, and enhancing overall effectiveness in expressing information.

By focusing on these strategies, individuals can significantly enhance their handwriting legibility, leading to better communication, academic success, and professional efficiency. Ultimately, clear and legible handwriting fosters confidence and ensures that written messages are delivered correctly and successfully.

UPPER CASE LETTER

INTRODUCTION:

Uppercase letters, commonly referred to as capital letters, are essential for written communication. In typography, they are more pronounced visually and give the text more structure than lowercase letters.

A B C D E F G H I J

K L M N O P Q R S T

U V W X Y Z

TWO TYPE LETTERS:

Upper Case Manuscript:

Block letters created without connecting strokes are which define manuscript or print style. Every letter is unique and simple to recognize. It is commonly taught in schools as the initial handwriting style for children. This is often introduced in kindergarten or preschool when children are around 4 to 5 years old. They start by learning to print uppercase letters individually.

Upper Case Cursive:

Cursive writing is a style where letters are joined together in a flowing manner. For cursive handwriting, it is necessary to move the pencil with a dynamic pencil grasp. While cursive is less common in everyday writing compared to manuscripts. After mastering the uppercase letters, children typically learn lowercase manuscript letters. This usually happens around the ages of 5 to 6, in kindergarten or first grade.

FOUNDATION SKILLS:

Understanding

Execution

Spacing

Punctuation

Capitalization guidelines

Uniformity

Proofreading

- **Understanding:** It is important to be able to identify uppercase letters in a variety of typefaces and styles. This means that one must be aware of the forms and unique qualities of every letter.
- **Execution:** Mastering the strokes and sequence are needed to construct the upper case letters accurately which is essential for proficient writing. Practicing the proper letter formation aids in developing consistency and legibility.
- **Spacing:** Grasping the appropriate spacing between upper case letters within words and between words is vital for readability and visual appeal in writing.

- **Punctuation:** Knowing when to use upper case letters alongside punctuation marks, such as, at the beginning of sentences, after periods, and in abbreviations, is critical for conveying meaning accurately.
- **Capitalization guidelines:** Understanding the rules of capitalization, including when to capitalize proper nouns, titles, acronyms, and the first letter of each sentence, is fundamental for adhering to standard language conventions.
- **Uniformity:** Consistently applying upper case letters according to established rules and conventions help to maintain clarity and professionalism in written communication.
- **Proofreading:** Developing the ability to proofread written work for capitalization errors ensures accuracy and refinement in final drafts.

COMMON PROBLEMS ENCOUNTERED IN UPPERCASE MANUSCRIPT AND CURSIVE WRITING:

Fine motor skill development

Lack of exposure or practice

Learning differences

Visual perception issues

Instructional methods

Lack of interest or engagement

Environmental factors

- **Fine motor skills development:** The child may struggle with controlling hand movements necessary for forming upper case letters accurately. Fine motor skills are crucial for precise letter formation, and difficulties in this area can hinder the child's ability to write upper case letters.

- **Lack of exposure or practice:** If the child does not have sufficient exposure to upper case letters or does not practice writing them regularly, they may struggle with letter formation and recognition. Regular practice is essential for mastering any skill, including writing upper case letters.
- **Learning differences or disabilities:** Conditions such as Dysgraphia, Dyslexia, or Developmental Coordination Disorder can impact a child's ability to write effectively, including forming upper case letters. These conditions may affect motor control, visual processing, and cognitive skills necessary for letter formation.
- **Visual perception issues:** Difficulties in perceiving and understanding the shapes and forms of letters can impede a child's ability to write upper case letters properly. Visual perception issues may affect the child's ability to distinguish between different letters and accurately replicate their shapes.
- **Instructional methods**: Ineffective teaching methods or a mismatch between the child's learning style and teaching techniques can hinder their ability to grasp and execute upper case letter writing. The child may require alternative instructional approaches that cater to their individual needs and learning preferences.
- **Lack of interest or engagement:** Some children may lack motivation or interest in practicing upper case letters, which can affect their progress in this skill. Without intrinsic or extrinsic motivation, the child may not invest the necessary effort to improve their letter formation abilities.
- **Environmental factors:** Distractions, discomfort, or stress in the learning environment can impact a child's focus and ability to learn and practice writing upper case letters effectively. A supportive and conducive learning environment is essential for promoting concentration and engagement in writing practice.

INTERVENTION FOR UPPER CASE MANUSCRIPT LETTER

- Phonic songs ABC's – memory
- Teaching position using rhymes - front, back, up, down etc
- Build a letter using rice/ sticks/ dhals etc. – letter formation, memory
- Tracing capital letter in kinetic sand - letter formation, memory, position, size
- Marker tracing activity
- Practicing corner letters eg. F, E, N, H, I etc
- Practicing centre letters eg. C, O, G, S, etc
- Wood pieces chart activity - arranging the capital letter using cardboard
- Slate chalkboard activity with lines – Letter formation activity, orientation, size.
- Copying the shapes and coloring activity
- Wide double line writing practice
- Read, color and draw activity – letters
- Ball catch - right left discrimination activity
- Writing on wall/ air – tracing activity
- Letter building toy activity
- Alphabet rhymes linking with words – Eg. CAT
- Spatial orientation activity
- Practicing corner word Eg. HEN, INK etc
- Practicing center word Eg. DOG, CUP etc
- Spelling tracing activity
- Read, color, and draw activity – words
- Phonic cup literacy game
- Build a keyboard activity with words
- Slate chalkboard activity with lines – word writing
- Reading a letter story
- Double line writing

INTERVENTION FOR UPPER CASE CURSIVE LETTER:

- **Dynamic pencil grasp**: Emphasize the importance of a dynamic pencil grasp for cursive handwriting. Encourage students to move the pencil smoothly along the lines of words.
- **Pre-cursive activities**: Engage students in pre-cursive activities and exercises to enhance dexterity required for cursive letters. These activities can include tracing patterns, shapes, or simple cursive strokes.
- **Alphabet and name writing**: Introduce students to cursive writing by teaching them to write the alphabet and their names in cursive. This typically aligns with the developmental stage around second grade, when fine motor skills are sufficiently developed.
- **Fine motor skill development**: Highlight the importance of fine motor skill development, which typically peaks around 7-8 years old. Encourage activities that promote pencil control, precision, and manipulation of the thumb and intrinsic hand muscles.
- **Visual reference**: Utilize cursive handwriting fonts as visual references for students. Show them examples of well-formed cursive letters to serve as a model for their own handwriting. Start with pre-cursive fonts to help students grasp the basic cursive letter forms before progressing to more complex styles.

RULES OF CURSIVE WRITING:

- Ensure all similar letters are in same height.
- Begin all small letters from the top.
- Form good handwriting using a pattern of ovals and parallel lines.
- Capital letters in cursive writing should generally not exceed the height of other letters.
- Make sure all downward strokes of letters are parallel.

Activity 1: Using a pencil, draw waves, angles, bumps, and loops on the page. Students can then trace these lines with highlighters or colored marker

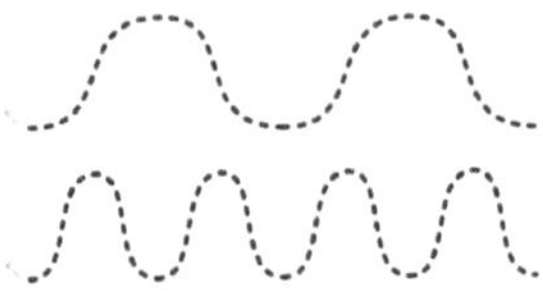

WAVES

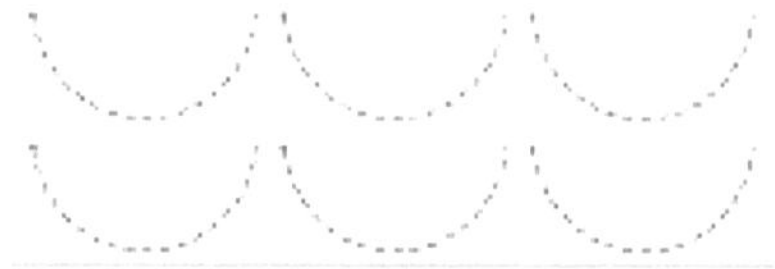

BUMPS

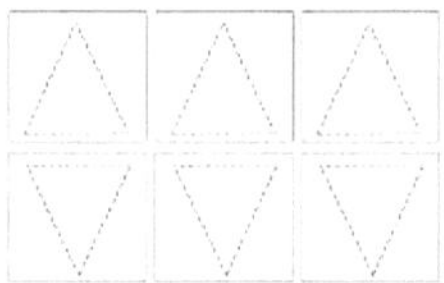

ANGLES

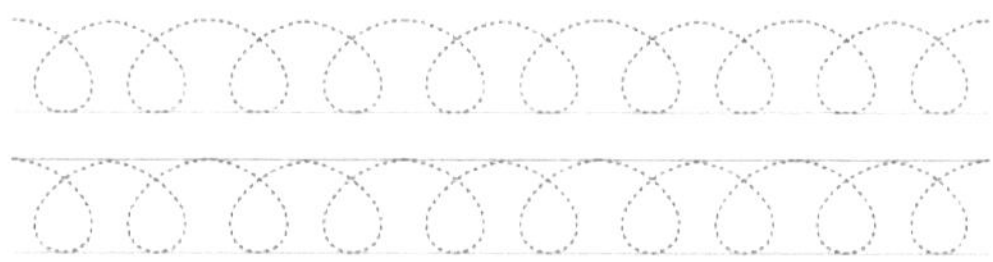

LOOPS

Activity 2: Draw a wave, curve, and a series of bumps or loops across a page with a pen. Students can trace the lines with glue and, once it hardens, trace the glue line with their fingers.

Activity 3: Draw a wave, curve, and a series of bumps or loops and trace them with a finger in a sensory tray.

Activity 4: Use wikki stix to build fine motor strength and dexterity. Stick the ends of the bendable, sticky pieces together to create a long strand. Use this strand to copy and create loops, cursive "c's," bumps, or angles.

Activity 5: Form and copy curves and spikes using jump ropes. Arrange several lines for the letter "w" or create bends by tying or placing the colourful jump ropes end to end on the floor.

Activity 6: Build cursive lines with craft pom poms. Have children copy or trace curves, loops, angles, or bumps with glue, then press the pom poms into the glue lines. This activity enhances fine motor skills and visual motor coordination.

Activity 7: Teach upper case cursive letters in the following order using worksheets: A, C, O, U, V, W, X, Y, Z, P, R, B, H, K, N, M, I, J, E, L, I, J, Q.

SUMMARY:

Uppercase letters play a vital role in written communication, marking emphasis, proper nouns, and the beginning of sentences. They come in two styles: manuscript (block letters) and cursive. Key foundation skills for writing uppercase letters include comprehension, execution, spacing, punctuation, capitalization rules, and uniformity. These skills are essential for mastering uppercase writing.

LOWER CASE LETTER

INTRODUCTION:

In the domain of handwriting, mastering lowercase letters is fundamental to effective communication and academic performance. This chapter explores into the shades of lowercase writing, encompassing both manuscript and cursive styles, through an exploration of developmental foundation skills, common problems, and intervention strategies for lowercase writing. The Occupational Therapist, educators, parents, and practitioners can gain valuable insights into promoting proficient lowercase writing skills in learners. Lowercase writing refers to the formation of small letters in contrast to uppercase or capital letters within an alphabetic writing system.

a b c d e f g h i j k l m

n o p q r s t u v w x y z

SIGNIFICANCE OF LOWERCASE WRITING:

Fluency and legibility of handwriting have a big impact on academic performance. The ability to write in lowercase is correlated with reading comprehension and general literacy.

Writing in lowercase helps with cognitive functions like spelling and letter identification.

COMPONENTS OF LOWERCASE WRITING

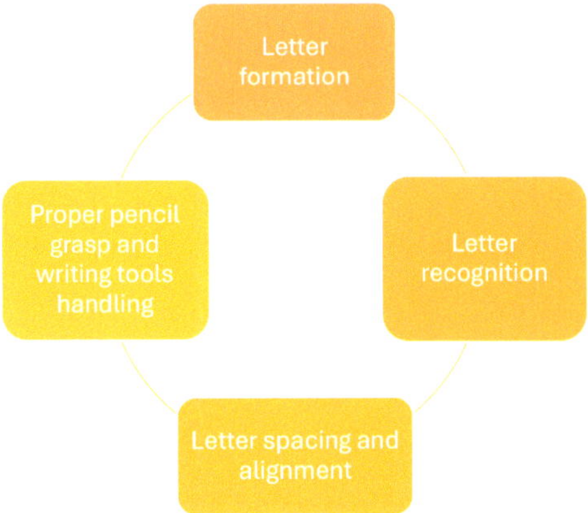

DIFFERENCES BETWEEN MANUSCRIPT AND CURSIVE LOWERCASE WRITING:

Aspect	Manuscript lowercase writing	Cursive lowercase writing
Letter formation	Letters are typically formed individually with distinct strokes	Letters are connected within words, often with continuous strokes
Stroke complexity	Generally simpler strokes, with clear separation between letters	More intricate strokes, with continuous flow between adjacent letters
Speed	Typically, slower due to individual letter formation	Potentially faster due to continuous writing without lifting the pen
Legibility	May vary based on consistency in letter formation and spacing	Legibility may improve with practice and fluidity in cursive writing
Instructional emphasis	Commonly taught in early childhood education as foundational skills	Historically taught in later grades or as a supplemental skill

FOUNDATION SKILLS IN LOWERCASE WRITING ACQUISITION:

- **Fine motor coordination**-The ability to coordinate small muscle movements, particularly in the hands and fingers, essential for precise letter formation.
- **Eye - hand Coordination**-The coordination between visual input and physical actions, crucial for controlling the movement of writing utensils and forming letters accurately.
- **Pencil grasp**-The way a child holds and controls a pencil or writing implementation, influencing the ease and precision of handwriting.
- **Letter recognition**-The ability to visually identify and discriminate between the lowercase letters, laying the foundation for accurate letter formation.
- **Spatial awareness**-Understanding and manipulating spatial relationships between letters, words, and lines on a page, ensuring proper spacing and alignment.
- **Visual perception**-The ability to interpret and make sense of visual stimuli, including letter shapes and orientations, essential for accurate letter formation.
- **Sequential memory**-Remembering the sequence of strokes required to form letters, aiding in the development of fluent and automatic handwriting.
- **Sensory integration**-The process of combining sensory information from multiple sources to produce a coordinated response, influencing handwriting fluency and legibility.

COMMON PROBLEMS ENCOUNTERED IN LOWERCASE MANUSCRIPT AND CURSIVE WRITING:

- **Letter reversals**-Difficulty distinguishing between mirror-image letters, such as b and d, p and q, leading to confusion in letter formation.

- **Letter formation inconsistencies**-Irregular or inconsistent formation of lowercase letters, resulting in illegible handwriting and difficulty in maintaining uniformity.
- **Spatial awareness problems**-Challenges with spacing between letters and words, leading to overcrowded or unevenly spaced writing that affects readability.
- **Poor line alignment** -Difficulty maintaining letters within designated lines, resulting in writing that drifts upwards, downwards, or across the page.
- **Slow writing speed**-Writing at a slower pace than peers, impacting productivity and fluency in written expression
- **Lack of pencil control** -Difficulty controlling the pencil or writing implementation, leading to shaky or erratic letter formation
- **Pencil grip issues** -Holding the pencil or writing tools improperly, leading to musculoskeletal discomfort, fatigue, or inefficient letter formation.
- **Overly large or small letter size** -Inconsistent letter sizing, resulting in letters that are disproportionately large or small compared to standard guidelines

EFFECTIVE INSTRUCTIONAL STRATEGIES FOR LOWERCASE WRITING:

- Incorporating multiple sensory modalities, such as tactile, visual, and auditory cues, to engage learners in the process of letter formation.
- Using rhymes, chants, and songs that correspond to the strokes and shapes of lowercase letters to reinforce letter formation through auditory repetition.
- Providing structured practice activities and worksheets that guide children through the step-by-step process of forming lowercase letters.
- Demonstrating letter formation for manuscript and cursive letters using clear and explicit visual models, such as letter

cards or writing guides, to provide concrete examples for learners.

- Gradually increasing the complexity of writing tasks and providing support as needed, such as by starting with tracing activities and progressing to independent writing.
- Promote regular and consistent practice of cursive writing skills, allocating dedicated time for handwriting instruction and reinforcement.
- Provide personalized feedback and corrective guidance to address specific challenges and errors in cursive letter formation.

INTERVENTION STRATEGIES TO ENHANCE LOWERCASE WRITING SKILLS:

- **Visual - motor integration exercises**: Incorporate activities that promote visual-motor integration, such as dot-to-dot tracing, mazes, and copying shapes or patterns, to enhance coordination between visual input and motor output.
- **Visual perceptual training activities**: Incorporate visual perceptual training exercises, such as visual scanning activities, form constancy tasks, and figure-ground discrimination, to enhance visual processing skills relevant to handwriting.
- **Environmental modifications**: Make environmental modifications to optimize the writing environment, such as adjusting desk height, providing ergonomic seating, and minimizing musculoskeletal discomforts and distractions.
- **Hand strengthening activities**: Implement activities using play dough, stress ball, theraputty, hand exercise balls and finger resistance bands targeting hand and finger muscles to improve grip strength and fine motor control necessary for precise writing movements.

- **Sandpaper letters**: Children trace letters carved on sandpaper with their fingers, promoting tactile and kinesthetic processing to promote letter formation.
- **Sand tray writing**: Children practices writing lowercase letters in a tray filled with sand, providing tactile feedback, and reinforcing letter formation.
- **Finger tracing**: Trace letters using their fingers on various textured surfaces, such as textured cards or sand trays, to enhance kinesthetic feedback
- **Air writing**: Practice forming letters in the air with their fingers, focusing on proper letter formation and stroke sequence. Children practice forming cursive letters in the air with their fingers while incorporating full-body movements, such as arm circles or leg kicks, to reinforce in learning letter shapes.
- **Sensory gel bags**: Children use their fingers to trace letters drawn on gel-filled bags, providing visual, tactile, and proprioceptive feedback
- **Finger painting letters:** Start with finger painting on a large sheet of paper. This tactile activity helps develop number recognition, finger strength and control of hand movements. Gradually transition to using a paintbrush or crayons.
- **Chalkboard or whiteboard writing**: Children practice writing letters on a chalkboard or whiteboard, providing auditory, visual, and kinesthetic feedback.
- **Playdough letter formation**: Children shapes playdough into letter forms, strengthening hand muscles and providing tactile and kinesthetic input.
- **Q-tip letter writing:** Start with large, simple letters for students to trace with Q-tip. Gradually reduce the size of the letters and increase the complexity. This Q-tip letter tracing activity is a great way for toddlers to learn the letters of the alphabet as well as begin writing.

- **Dot-to-dot activity:** Provide dot-to-dot worksheets that children can connect. Start with fewer dots and gradually increase the number of dots for more challenging tracing activity.
- **Constructing letters with lines and curves:** Constructing letters with lines and curves is an effective readiness skill for number writing and it is an incredibly fun activity.
- **Pencil control activities:** Begin with basic pencil control such as drawing straight lines, curves, and shapes. Gradually increase the complexity of the shapes and lines.
- **Modified paper and writing tools**: Provide modified paper with raised lines, colored lines, or highlighted spacing to assist individuals with maintaining proper letter size, spacing, and alignment. Adapted writing tools like pencil grips, adapted pencils with built-up grips or weighted ends can be used.
- **Spacing guides and paper templates**: Provide visual cues, such as raised lines or colored blocks, to assist students in maintaining consistent spacing between letters and words.
- **Letter collage creation activity**: Make the children cut out letters from magazines or newspapers to create collages. This activity helps them recognize and identify letters while also practicing fine motor skills.
- **Letter formation with nature**: Take children on a nature walk and collect natural materials like sticks, leaves, or rocks. Use these items to form letters on the ground, combining outdoor exploration with handwriting practice.
- **Musical letter writing**: Play upbeat music and make the children to write letters to the rhythm of the music. This activity promotes motor coordination and letter formation while adding an element of fun.
- **Cursive treasure hunt**: Hide laminated cursive letters around the room or outdoors. Children search for the letters and trace them with their fingers or write them down as they find them.

- **Cursive relay race**: Divide children into teams and set up a relay race where they must write cursive letters on a whiteboard or chalkboard before passing the marker to the next teammate. This activity adds a competitive element to cursive writing practice.
- **Cursive handwriting olympics:** Create stations with different cursive writing challenges, such as tracing, writing on a vertical surface, or writing with their non-dominant hand. Children rotate through the stations and earn medals or awards for completing each challenge.
- **Cursive secret messages**: Write messages in cursive on paper using invisible ink (lemon juice) or white crayon. Children reveal the hidden messages by painting over the paper with watercolor paint, adding an element of mystery and excitement to handwriting practice.
- **Handwriting obstacle course**: Set up an obstacle course with stations where students write specific lowercase letters in either manuscript or cursive before moving on to the next station.
- **Task - specific practice**: Provide task-specific practice focusing on repetitive writing tasks, gradually increasing in complexity and difficulty, to improve handwriting fluency and automaticity.
- **Offer corrective feedback**: Provide specific and constructive feedback on students cursive writing, addressing errors in letter formation, spacing, and overall legibility
- **Tailor made interventions**: Tailor made cursive writing instruction to meet the individual needs of students, offering additional support or accommodations as necessary.

SUMMARY:

In conclusion, mastering lowercase letter is a fundamental skill essential for academic success and everyday tasks. While individuals may encounter various challenges during the learning process, implementing targeted strategies and providing appropriate support can significantly enhance writing proficiency. By incorporating evidence-based practices, collaborating with educators, parents, and other professionals, and addressing specific challenges with practical tips and strategies, Occupational Therapists can effectively facilitate lowercase writing development in learners of all ages. Through ongoing assessment, monitoring, and adjustment of intervention strategies, Occupational Therapists play a vital role in promoting successful handwriting skills and empowering individuals.

UPPER CASE AND LOWER CASE LETTERS

CURSIVE AND MANUSCRIPT LETTERS

Aa Bb Cc Dd Ee Ff
Gg Hh Ii Jj Kk Ll
Mm Nn Oo Pp Qq
Rr Ss Tt Uu Vv Ww
Xx Yy Zz

Aa Bb Cc Dd Ee Ff Gg
Hh Ii Jj Kk Ll Mm Nn
Oo Pp Qq Rr Ss Tt Uu
Vv Ww Xx Yy Zz

COPYING

Copying is a common handwriting technique used to improve letter formation, which is an important component of legibility. Copying is the ability to reproduce numerals, letters, and words using a similar script model either manuscript to manuscript or cursive to cursive. Copying text quickly and accurately is useful in both school and everyday life.

- Near Point Copy
- Far Point Copy

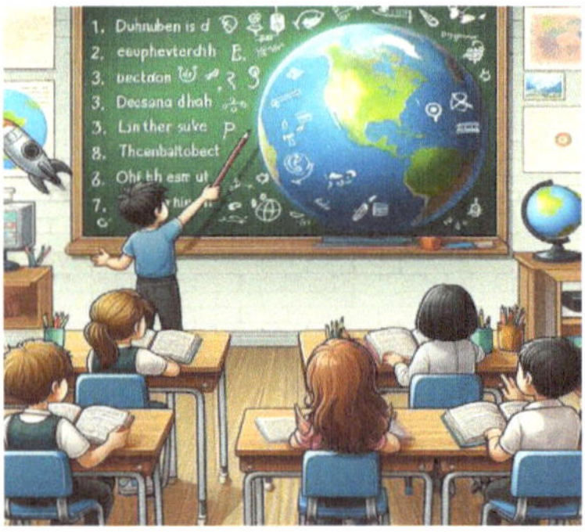

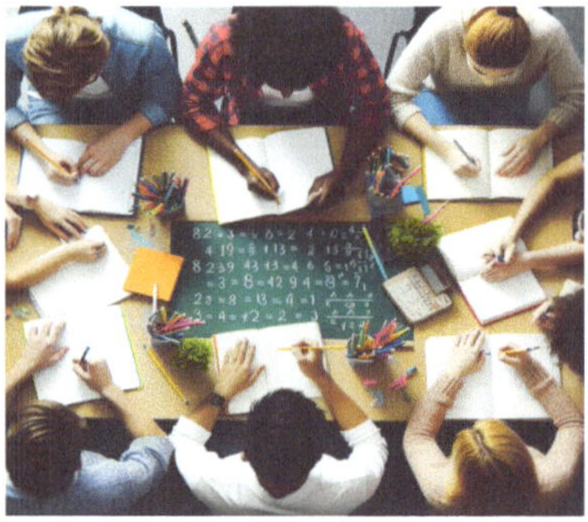

NEAR POINT COPYING

Introduction:

Near point copying is a visual function test that assesses a person's ability and evaluates the accuracy and efficiency of copying written or printed material at close range, usually within arm's length. It evaluates several aspects of visual perception, including visual acuity, accommodation, convergence, and visual-motor integration.

Near-point copying tasks are frequently used in optometric evaluations to assess visual function and identify abnormalities or deficiencies in visual processing and coordination. Near-point copying is the process of reproducing letters or words from a nearby model, typically on the same page or horizontal writing surface. Near point copying is a steppingstone to independent writing. Copying is an excellent way to learn to draw and write, while focusing directly on visual and fine motor skills.

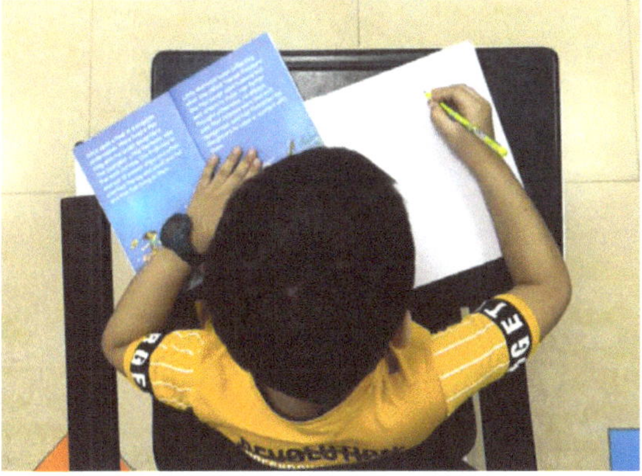

VISUAL PERCEPTION SKILLS:

Visual perceptual skills are those abilities that allow the children to make sense of what they visually see. Visual perceptual abilities are required for everything from navigating our environment to reading, writing, and manipulating objects. Visual perception is a complex combination of skills. The visual perceptual skills must work together in order to use visual information to generate responses or react with functional abilities such as movement or processing. Handwriting, including word copying, requires strong visual perceptual skills. Activities such as reading, writing, cutting, copying from the board, puzzles, object location, playground navigation, and eye-hand coordination involve visual perception skill.

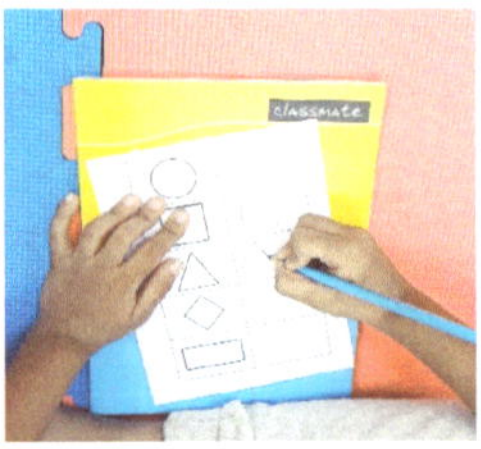
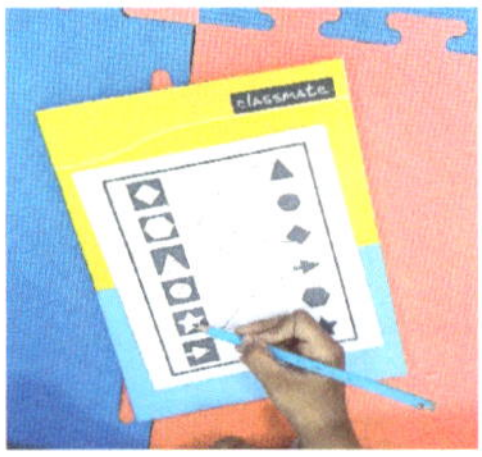
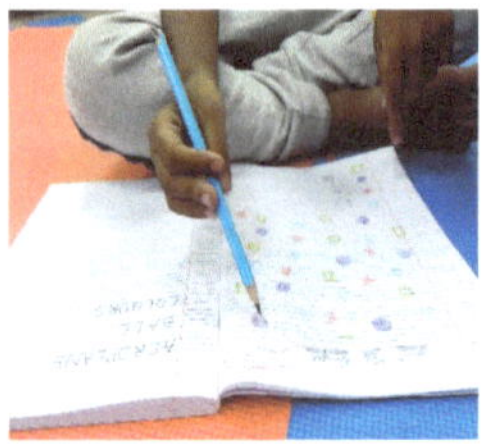
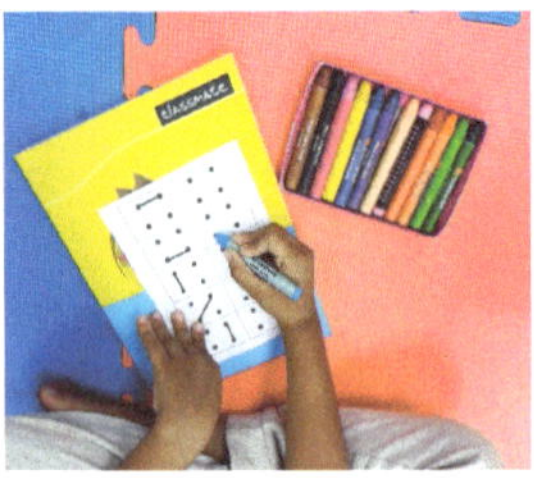
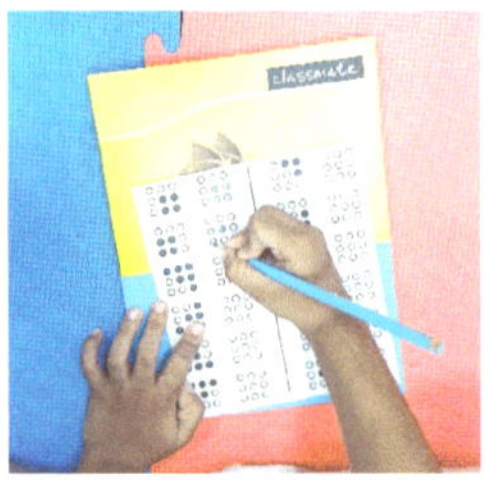

VISUAL PERCEPTION SKILLS INVOLVED IN NEAR POINT COPYING ARE:

1. Discrimination
2. Memory
3. Spatial relationships
4. Form constancy
5. Sequential memory
6. Motor integration
7. Attention and concentration
8. Scanning and tracking
9. Figure-ground discrimination
10. Closure

1. VISUAL DISCRIMINATION:

Near point copying necessitates an accurate perception and interpretation of visual information. Visual discrimination is the ability to recognize similarities and differences in shapes, sizes, colors, objects, and patterns. Visual discrimination is particularly important when learning to read and write. Children require adequate visual discrimination skills to perform properly in school and at home.

Occupational Therapy in visual discrimination refers to the ability to accurately perceive and distinguish between visual stimuli such as letters, numbers, shapes, and objects. This skill is essential for activities such as reading, writing, and identifying objects in the environment.

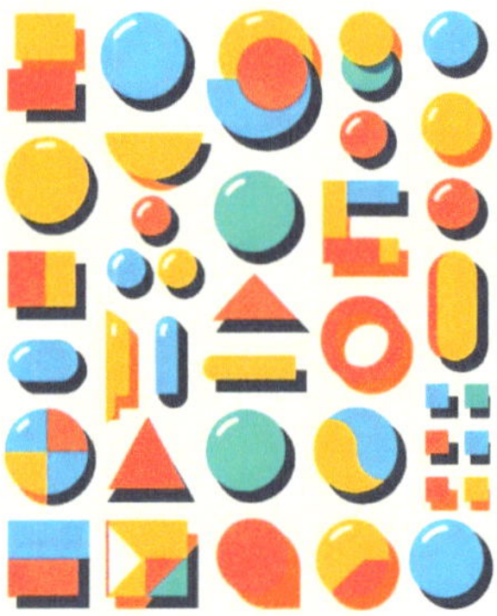

OCCUPATIONAL THERAPY IN VISUAL DISCRIMINATION:

Occupational Therapists evaluate an individual's visual discrimination abilities and design interventions to improve them. These interventions could include activities like matching games, sorting tasks, pattern recognition exercises, and visual scanning activities. Occupational Therapists help people to improve their overall functional performance and independence in everyday life by improving visual discrimination.

2. VISUAL MEMORY:

Near point copying usually includes remembering visual information. Visual memory refers to the ability to recall information received by the brain. This skill enables us to recall the appearance of a shape, symbol, object, or form, which is essential for learning and daily activities. Most academic tasks require visual memory, including reading, spelling, and copying from the board.

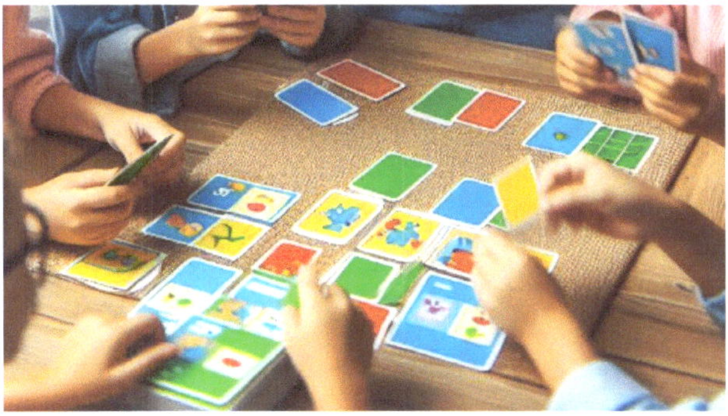

OCCUPATIONAL THERAPY IN VISUAL MEMORY:

Occupational Therapy in visual memory involves evaluating and improving an individual's ability to retain and recall visual information. The skill is essential for tasks such as following directions, remembering faces, and recognizing objects. Occupational Therapists evaluate an individual's abilities of visual memory and design interventions to improve them. Memory games, pattern recognition exercises, and strategies for improving visual information encoding and retrieval are some of the interventions available. Occupational Therapists assist people in improving their overall cognitive function and independence in everyday life by improving visual memory.

3. VISUAL SPATIAL RELATIONS:

Visual spatial relations is an important visual perceptual skill that is important for many functional tasks. Spatial relations allow the organization of the body in relation to objects or spatial awareness. This is an important part of spatial awareness in handwriting. A crucial aspect of visual spatial relations involves understanding laterality and directionality. Essentially, these terms relate to awareness of left-right orientation in the body and the capacity to recognize the left/right positioning of objects. Spatial relations also plays a vital role in near point copying skills, or accuracy of copying written work.

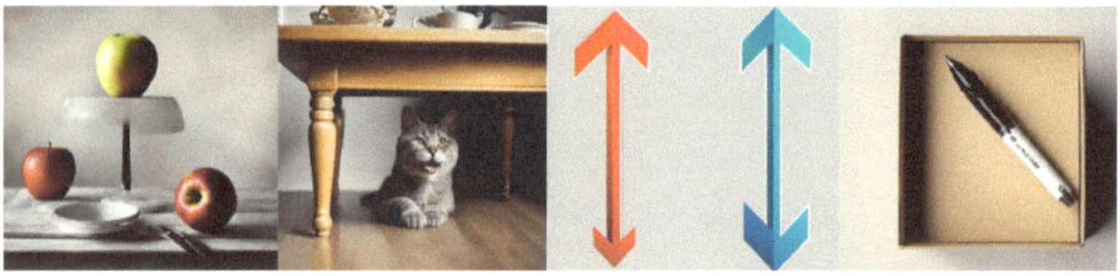

OCCUPATIONAL THERAPY IN VISUAL SPATIAL RELATIONS:

In Occupational Therapy for copying skills, visual spatial relations involve understanding the arrangement and spacing of visual elements when reproducing them from a model or reference material. Therapists usually works on improving these skills by helping individuals accurately perceive and replicate the size, shape, and spatial arrangement of letters, words, or images. Activities may include practicing copying tasks with attention to proper alignment, spacing, and proportion, as well as activities to enhance visual tracking and attention to detail. Strengthening visual spatial relations facilitates more accurate and efficient copying abilities.

4. VISUAL FORM CONSTANCY:

Visual form constancy is a visual perception skill that refers to the ability to recognize an object (the 'form') is still the same thing despite changes in orientation, direction, size, or distance. This ability encompasses a mixture of visual discrimination, visual memory, and visual perception of figure-ground relationships. It involves perceiving an object or shape as being consistent and unchanged even when viewed from different angles or in different contexts.

Visual form constancy is essential for refining near point copying skills, particularly in tasks requiring accurate reproduction of visual stimuli. This skill enables individuals to recognize and understand that a visual stimulus remains the same, regardless of variations in size, orientation, or position.

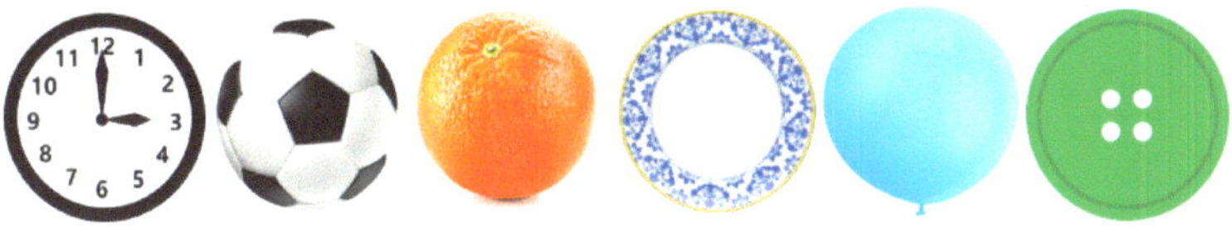

OCCUPATIONAL THERAPY IN VISUAL FORM CONSTANCY:

The Occupational Therapists utilizes the targeted interventions such as tracing exercises, matching tasks with varying sizes or orientations, and puzzles that require consistent identification of shapes or patterns. By strengthening visual form constancy, individuals can improve their ability to maintain consistent letter formations, sizes, and alignments when copying text or images from proximity references, ultimately enhancing overall accuracy and efficiency in near point copying tasks.

5. VISUAL SEQUENTIAL MEMORY:

Visual sequential memory refers to the capacity to recall visual information as received in the same sequential manner. It helps to pay attention in the order of objects, symbols and details. It is required for reading, spelling, math, printing and copying from the board.

Visual sequential memory plays a vital role in enhancing near point copying skills, particularly in handwriting tasks. This skill involves the ability to remember and accurately reproduce a sequence of visual stimuli in the proper order, which is essential for accurately copying the text or images from a model or reference material.

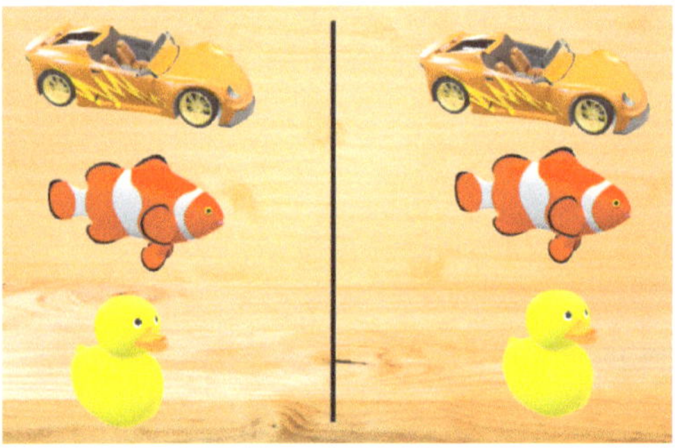

OCCUPATIONAL THERAPY IN VISUAL SEQUENTIAL MEMORY:

Occupational Therapists employ targeted interventions such as tracing activities, copying tasks with gradually increasing complexity, and memory games focusing on sequential patterns. By improving visual sequential memory, individuals can better retain and reproduce the order of letters, words, or shapes when copying, leading to improved accuracy, legibility, and efficiency in handwriting tasks.

6. VISUAL-MOTOR INTEGRATION:

Visual motor integration refers to the ability to interpret visual stimuli and respond with a motor action. Visual motor integration for Near copying skills refers to the coordination of visual perception and motor skills to accurately replicate written material or images presented at a close distance. In short, it is the ability to observe something and accurately reproduce it using hand movements. To properly reproduce the copied material, the individual must transform visual information into precise hand movements. This requires better eye - hand coordination, fine motor control and visual perceptual skills.

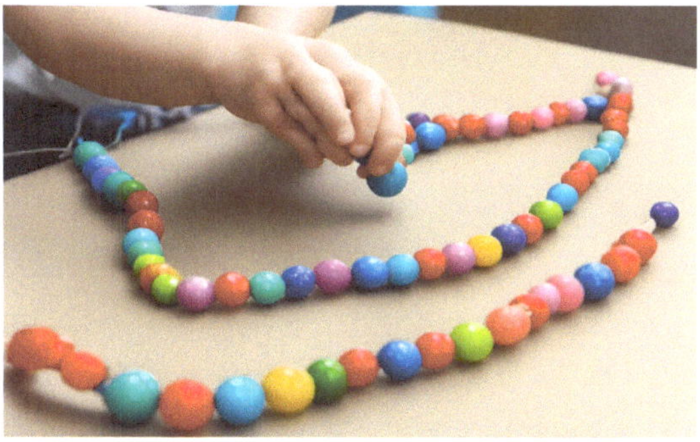

OCCUPATIONAL THERAPY IN VISUAL MOTOR INTEGRATION:

Occupational Therapy in visual-motor integration focuses on improving coordination between visual perception and motor skills. This includes the ability to interpret visual information and accurately coordinate hand movements to complete tasks efficiently. Occupational Therapists evaluate an individual's visual-motor integration skills and develop interventions to improve them. Tracing shapes, copying patterns, and practicing eye-hand coordination are some of the interventions that may be used. Occupational Therapists help people to improve their ability to engage in activities like handwriting, drawing, and other fine motor tasks, resulting in greater independence and participation in daily life.

7. VISUAL ATTENTION AND CONCENTRATION:

Visual attention and concentration in near point copying skills refer to the ability to focus and maintain attention on the model while accurately reproducing it. It requires providing attention to details and avoiding distractions throughout the copying process to ensure that the copied material is replicated precisely better visual attention and concentration skills are required to maintain accuracy and complete near point copying tasks efficiently. The individual must maintain focus on the model while reproducing it without errors.

OCCUPATIONAL THERAPY IN VISUAL ATTENTION AND CONCENTRATION:

Occupational Therapy in visual attention and concentration includes evaluating and improving a person's ability to maintain focus on visual tasks. This ability is necessary for activities such as reading, writing, and completing tasks that require sustained visual attention. Occupational Therapists evaluate a person's visual attention and concentration abilities and create interventions to improve these abilities. These interventions may include activities to improve visual scanning and attention to detail, as well as distraction-reduction strategies. Occupational Therapists help people improve their overall functional performance and participation in everyday activities by improving their visual attention and concentration.

8. VISUAL SCANNING AND TRACKING:

Visual scanning is the ability to use vision to observe in a systematic manner, such as top to bottom and left to right. A child needs to use visual scanning to avoid obstacles when navigating their environment. Smooth visual scanning is required for reading.

Visual tracking is defined as efficiently focusing on an object as it moves across a person's visual field. This skill is important for daily activities, including reading, writing, drawing, and playing.

OCCUPATIONAL THERAPY IN VISUAL SCANNING AND TRACKING:

In Occupational Therapy, visual scanning and tracking are integral for refining near point copying skills, particularly in tasks requiring individuals to efficiently locate and follow visual stimuli within proximity. Visual scanning involves the systematic exploration of visual information, enabling individuals to identify specific items or details within a given area, while visual tracking involves smoothly and accurately following a moving object or line of text with the eyes. Occupational Therapists utilize targeted interventions such as worksheets with grids of letters or words for scanning exercises, activities that require tracking a moving object or line while copying, and games that promote rapid and accurate visual scanning and tracking. By strengthening visual scanning and tracking, individuals can enhance their ability to quickly locate and accurately reproduce text or images from proximity references, leading to improved speed and precision in near point copying tasks.

9. VISUAL FIGURE-GROUND DISCRIMINATION:

Figure ground perception is the ability to filter the visual information that is not important so that you can focus on the required visual information. This allows to find detailed visual information even when it is part of a messy background. Visual figure ground perception allows to pick up on required visual information while ignoring extraneous visual information. Figure ground discrimination is important in copying words from the front of the room, reading specific information on the board in the front of the room, maintaining your visual attention for long periods of time, and finding objects in a particular place.

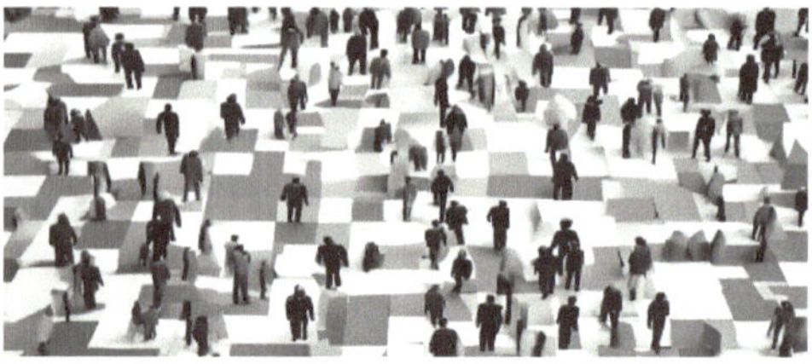

OCCUPATIONAL THERAPY IN VISUAL FIGURE GROUND DISCRIMINATION:

In Occupational Therapy, visual figure-ground discrimination is pivotal for honing near point copying skills, especially in tasks requiring individuals to distinguish a target object from its background or surrounding visual stimuli. This skill enables individuals to focus on and accurately reproduce specific elements of a visual stimulus while ignoring irrelevant background details. Occupational Therapists use specific interventions such as worksheets with contrasting backgrounds to highlight target letters or words, activities involving the identification of specific items within a cluttered visual field, and exercises that emphasize isolating relevant visual information from distractions. By strengthening visual figure-ground discrimination, individuals can enhance their ability to accurately perceive and reproduce text or images from proximity references, leading to improved precision and efficiency in near point copying tasks.

10. VISUAL CLOSURE:

Visual closure is a visual perceptual ability that enables individuals to recognize objects even when only partially visible. This skill is essential for identifying objects and mentally completing their visual representation before seeing the entire object. It plays a crucial role in rapid reading, fluent reading, and distinguishing differences between similar words.

OCCUPATIONAL THERAPY IN VISUAL CLOSURE:

In Occupational Therapy, visual closure plays a crucial role in refining near point copying skills, particularly in tasks requiring the ability to perceive complete visual stimuli from partial or fragmented information. This skill enables individuals to accurately recognize and reproduce entire letters, words, or shapes even when portions of the visual stimulus are obscured or incomplete. Occupational Therapists employ targeted interventions such as completing partial drawings or letters, puzzles requiring the identification of objects from incomplete patterns, and activities that encourage the visualization of whole forms from fragmented information. By strengthening visual closure, individuals can enhance their ability to copy text or images accurately and efficiently from proximity references, improving overall accuracy and proficiency in near point copying tasks.

FINE MOTOR CONTROL:

Fine motor control for near point copying skills includes precisely coordinating small muscle movements in the fingers, hands, and wrists to accurately reproduce written material or images presented at a close distance. Near point copying tasks require precise manipulation of writing utensils or tools to reproduce the copied material with clarity and accuracy. Individuals with strong fine motor control can maintain a steady hand, control the pressure applied on the writing tools, and perform controlled movements such as letter formation, spacing, and alignment. Furthermore, fine motor control enables the people to manage the intricate hand movements required for tasks like tracing lines, shapes, or small details.

OCCUPATIONAL THERAPY IN FINE MOTOR CONTROL:

Occupational Therapy in fine motor control focuses on improving hand and finger movement coordination and precision. This skill is required for activities like writing, buttoning clothes, and using utensils. Occupational Therapists evaluate an individual's fine motor control abilities and design interventions to improve them. These interventions may include finger exercises, hand strengthening activities, and tasks that necessitate precise hand movements, such as threading beads or using scissors. Occupational Therapists help people improve their ability to participate in daily activities and gain independence by improving their fine motor control.

SPEED AND EFFICIENCY:

Individuals with proficient near point copying skills can complete copying tasks efficiently, with minimal errors, and without exerting too much effort. Individuals speed and accuracy in copying written material or images can be improved through practice and skill development.

OCCUPATIONAL THERAPY IN SPEED AND EFFICIENCY:

Occupational Therapy for speed and efficiency in near point copying focuses on improving the ability to accurately replicate written material or images presented at a close distance in a reasonable time frame. This skill is essential for tasks like handwriting, which require individuals to produce legible and clear copies quickly. Occupational Therapists use a variety of techniques to improve speed and efficiency, including timed copying tasks, ergonomic positioning strategies, and feedback on efficient copying techniques. Individuals who improve their speed and efficiency in near point copying can complete tasks more quickly and effectively, ultimately improving their overall functional performance in activities requiring close visual attention and fine motor control.

ACTIVITIES TO IMPROVE NEAR POINT COPYING:

- Puzzles.
- Draw or paint pictures.
- Find as many things as you can see of a certain shape (circle, square, rectangle, triangle) in the room.
- Copy a sequence of physical actions performed by another person.
- Perform dot-to-dot pictures.
- Find the mistakes in "What's Wrong with this Picture?"
- Sort playing cards in different ways (color, suit, number), or use playing cards to find two with matching numbers.
- Solve mazes.
- Use tracing paper to trace and color simple pictures.
- Play flashlight chases. Engage in this activity by obtaining flashlights. Lie on the back into the floor and make the child to chase flashlight beam.
- Make the child to go through a page of print (according to reading level) and circle all the target letters or numbers.
- Use a slant board for reading.
- Ball games.
- Painting with marbles.
- Cup shuffle.

- Painting with a straw.
- Text tracking activity-read the first and last word.
- Moving the object like a pendulum.
- Flashlight tag - use laser pointer on a wall and watch the red dot while sweeping it across the wall, go up, down, left, right and diagonally.
- Read aloud-helps the eyes and brain to work together.
- Color pattern matching game.
- Fill the dot with colors.
- Hide and seek with toys.
- Scavenger hunt in a book-call out word that are used often such as the, and, who etc.
- Collecting and packing items for school bags.
- Games such as Simon Says.
- Sequencing games e.g. Recall a sequence of colored beads threaded onto a string, then conceal it from view and attempt to replicate it from memory.
- Copying body sequences e.g. 3 hops forward, 1 jump back.
- Tangram.
- Crawling under, over, and through objects without touching them.

SUMMARY:

Near point copying is a visual function test that assesses a person's ability to copy the written or printed material accurately and efficiently at close range. It evaluates various aspects of visual perception such as discrimination, memory, spatial relationships, form constancy, sequential memory, motor integration, attention, concentration, scanning and tracking, figure ground discrimination and closure.

FAR POINT COPYING

WHAT IS FAR POINT COPYING?

The term "**Far Point Copying**" is usually referred to a visual motor skill assessed in early childhood. It is about the ability to accurately copy or trace objects, shapes, and letters from a distance. In this context, **"Far Point"** indicates that the child is copying from a visual stimulus placed at a distance rather than up close. Visual motor integration skills, which are involved in coordinating visual perception with eye-hand coordination for preschoolers, are frequently evaluated. The ability to visually perceive an object or shape from a distance and then accurately reproduce it on paper or the surface shall be assessed when performing far point copying tasks. Such skills are essential for a variety of activities in young children's education, e.g. the development of basic motor skills, learning to read letters and numbers or participating in visual arts and crafts activity. Difficulty with far point copying may indicate challenges with visual perception, spatial awareness, or fine motor coordination, which might warrant further assessment or intervention to support the child's development.

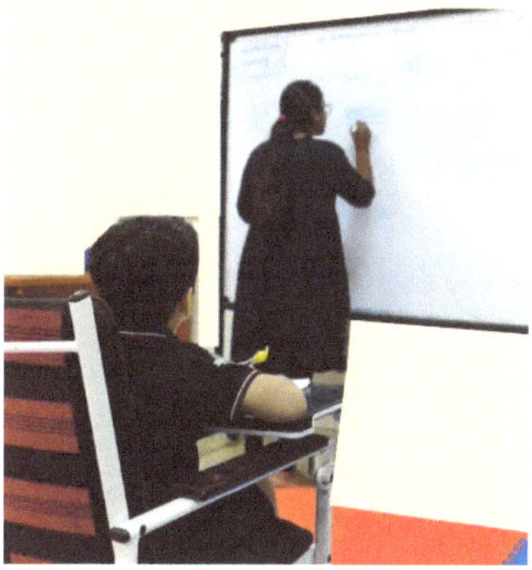

SKILLS FOR FAR POINT COPYING INCLUDES:

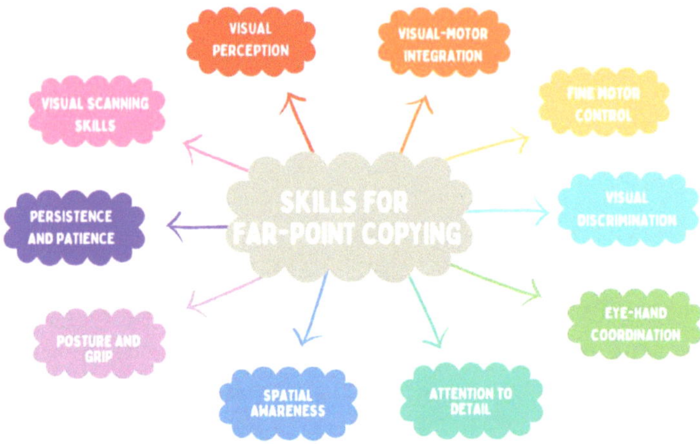

1. VISUAL PERCEPTION

Visual perception is the process of interpreting visual stimuli and giving them meanings and connotations. Visual perception is the ability to interpret visual information from the surroundings and make sense of what is seen.

Visual Discrimination

Visual discrimination is the capacity to notice differences and classify objects, symbols, or shapes. These distinctions can be based on color, position, form, pattern, texture, and size. Essentially, the eyes receive environmental input, which various cells then detect and send as signals to the brain. For visual discrimination, the visual cortex in the occipital lobe is key to identifying the shape and orientation of objects. The primary visual cortex contains three types of cells — simple, complex, and hypercomplex that progressively enhance the ability to respond to motion and linearity.

Visual Closure

Visual closure is the ability to perceive and recognize objects, shapes, features, or symbols from incomplete or degraded visual stimuli. This skill demonstrates the human capacity to fill in missing information from incomplete sensory input to form a meaningful perception.

Visual Figure-Ground

Figure-ground refers to the segmentation of visual information into objects and their surrounding backgrounds, which provides structure for visual attention.

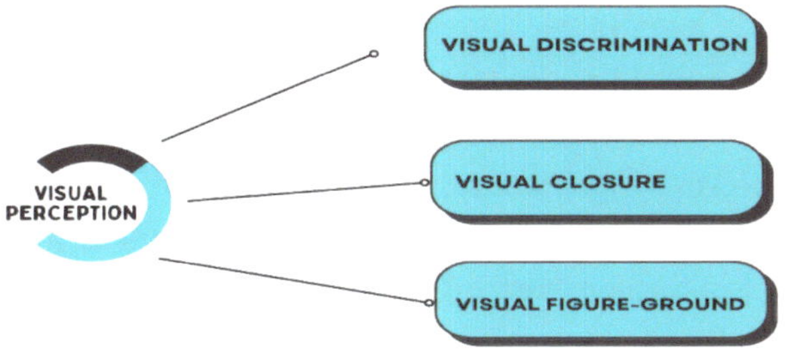

2.VISUAL MOTOR INTEGRATION

Visual-Motor Integration (VMI) is the ability to use input from the visual perceptive system—including visual acuity, accommodation, binocular fusion, stereopsis, and convergence/divergence—to coordinate fine motor skills. These skills involve the smaller muscles of the wrist and hand, encompassing dexterity, precision, coordination, and manual control. VMI is essential for many everyday activities such as handwriting, drawing, catching a ball, dressing, eating, and driving.

There are two types of VMI:

- **Constructional VMI:** Involves tasks like using blocks to build a 3D shape.

- **Graphomotor VMI:** Involves paper and pencil tasks, such as drawing lines to form geometric shapes.

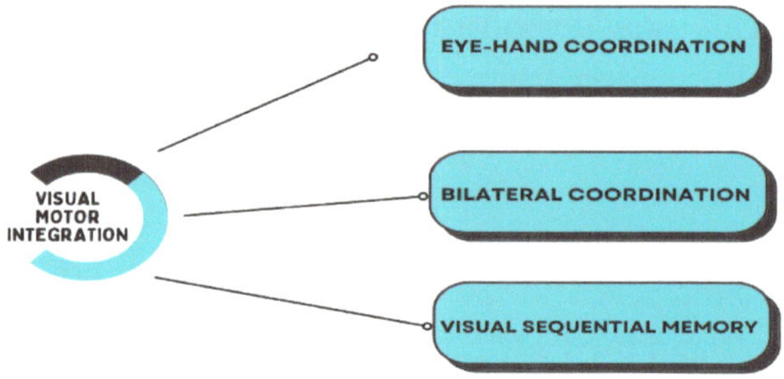

Eye-Hand Coordination

Eye–hand coordination refers to the ability to produce goal-oriented hand actions that are guided by visual information from the eyes. Good coordination between the sensory visual system and the musculoskeletal system is required for efficient and effective human function during interaction with the nearby environment.

Bilateral Coordination

Bilateral integration is the ability to use information from both sides of the body to coordinate efficient movement. Bilateral coordination involves using both hands for simultaneous and alternating movements. Working on bilateral coordination helps to:

- Promote crossing the midline for smooth writing.
- Stabilize the paper while writing.
- Coordinate typing with both hands instead of finger pecking.

Visual Sequential Memory

Visual sequential memory refers to the cognitive ability to remember and recall a sequence of visual information in the order it was presented. It involves the encoding, storage, and retrieval of visual information in a specific sequence. This type of memory is crucial for various everyday tasks such as reading, following instructions, solving puzzles, and navigating spatial environments. In essence, visual sequential memory enables individuals to remember the order of visual elements, such as numbers, letters, shapes, or objects, and to reproduce or recall them in the correct sequence. It plays a significant role in academic performance, particularly in subjects like mathematics, where the ability to remember the sequence of numerical operations is essential, and in language acquisition, where recalling the order of letters is fundamental for reading and writing. Additionally, it is relevant in activities like following directions, playing musical instruments, and sports that require precise execution of sequences of movements.

3. FINE MOTOR CONTROL

Fine motor skills involve the coordination of spatio-temporal processing, visuomotor integration, strength control, perceptual, and cognitive abilities. These interconnected skills exemplify networked neuromotor development. Different graphomotor tasks, like writing and drawing, engage both shared and unique neural circuits in the motor and posterior parietal regions. Drawing activates a ventral pathway responsible for spatial orientation, while writing engages a dorsal pathway that controls letter formation.

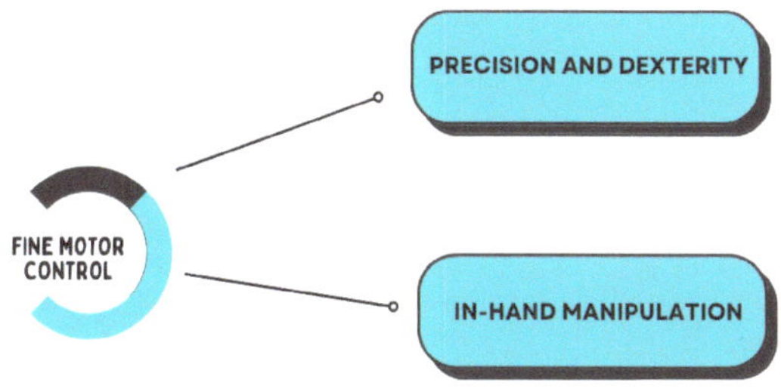

Precision and Dexterity

Stable precision grips, using the fingertips, are fundamental to human hand dexterity. This grip style involves the precise and stable application of fingertip forces, with the fingers remaining relatively stationary while the fingertips exert force. The development of stable precision grips was crucial in the evolution of hand dexterity.

In-Hand Manipulation

In-Hand Manipulation refers to the ability to manipulate objects within one hand, using various movements such as rotation, translation, and shifting. This skill is essential for tasks like writing, drawing, buttoning, and manipulating small objects. It involves precise coordination of the fingers and hand muscles to perform intricate movements efficiently.

4. ATTENTION TO DETAILS

Attention optimizes the processing resources of the individual by enhancing the information of interest at a given moment and inhibiting the stimuli, identified as task-irrelevant at that time. It can operate either endogenously, driven by the goals of the perceiver (e.g., I am looking for a friend in a crowd of people) or exogenously, by the stimulus properties (e.g., a flashing light captures my attention).

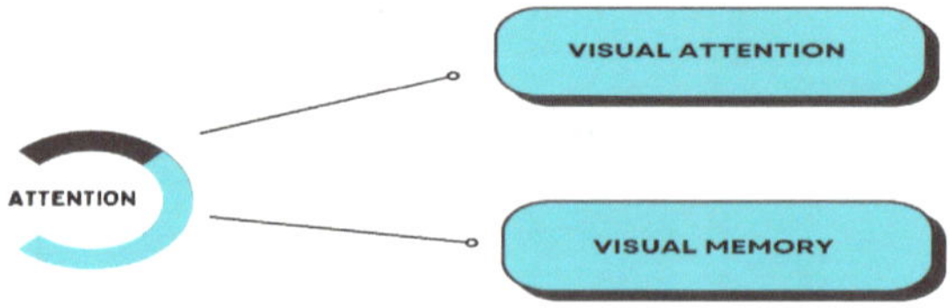

Visual Attention

Visual attention is a crucial aspect of higher-level cognition, especially in humans, for whom vision is the primary sense. It refers to cognitive processes that enable us to selectively process the vast amount of information the people encounter daily. Due to the limitations of the perceptual system, focusing on specific aspects of the visual field allows us to prioritize relevant information and disregard irrelevant details.

Visual Memory

Visual memory involves encoding visual stimuli into memory, retaining these mental representations over time, and accurately recalling them when needed. This type of memory is essential for tasks such as reading, problem-solving, spatial navigation, and artistic expression.

5. SPATIAL AWARENESS

Spatial awareness encompasses the ability to comprehend and perceive one's surroundings, including the relationships between objects, oneself, and the environment. It involves understanding distances, directions, shapes, and sizes within physical spaces. Spatial awareness relies on cognitive skills such as perception, memory, and reasoning, enabling individuals to mentally visualize and manipulate spatial information effectively.

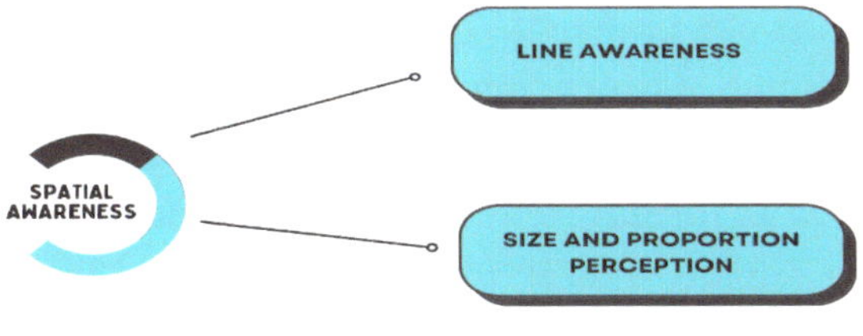

Line Awareness

Line awareness in handwriting refers to the ability to write consistently and accurately along a straight line or baseline. It involves maintaining proper alignment of letters, words, and sentences on a page, ensuring legibility and neatness in handwriting. Individuals with good line awareness can control the spacing and alignment of their writing, resulting in well-organized and visually appealing text.

Size and Proportion perception

Size and proportion perception in handwriting refers to the ability to maintain consistent letter sizes and proportions throughout written text. It involves accurately judging the relative sizes of individual letters, words, and spaces between them to ensure uniformity and legibility. Individuals with good size and proportion perception in handwriting can produce text that is visually balanced and well-proportioned, enhancing readability and aesthetics.

6. POSTURE AND GRIP

Posture and grip in handwriting refers to the physical positioning of the body and the way the writing instrument is held while writing. Posture involves the alignment of the body, particularly the trunk, shoulders, and arms, to provide stability and support during writing. Grip refers to the way an individual holds the writing instrument, including the finger position and pressure exerted on the pen or pencil.

An optimal posture and grip in handwriting facilitate efficient and comfortable writing, allowing for greater control and precision in forming letters and words. Poor posture or grip can lead to fatigue, musculoskeletal discomfort, and decreased legibility in handwriting.

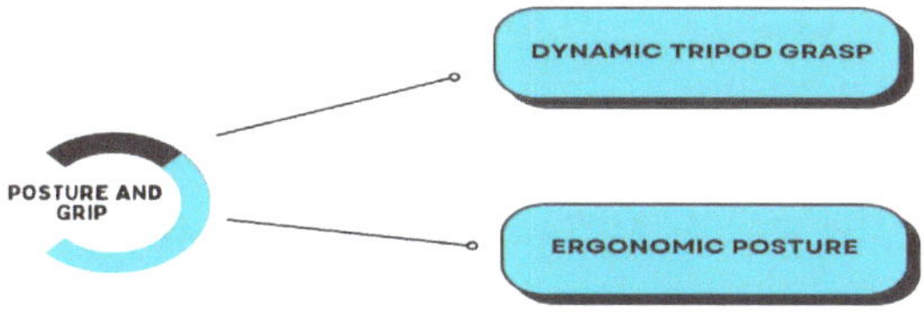

Dynamic Tripod Grasp

Dynamic tripod grasp in handwriting refers to a specific and efficient way of holding a writing instrument where the pen or pencil is held between the thumb and the index finger, with the middle finger providing support underneath. This grip allows for controlled and precise movement of the writing implement while minimizing strain and fatigue on the hand and fingers. The dynamic tripod grasp is characterized by a relaxed and comfortable hand position that promotes fluidity and legibility in handwriting.

Ergonomic Posture

Ergonomic posture in handwriting refers to the optimal body positioning and alignment that promotes comfort, efficiency, and safety during the act of writing. This includes proper positioning of the body, chair, desk, and writing surface to reduce strain on muscles and joints, alleviate discomfort, and minimize the risk of developing musculoskeletal disorders associated with prolonged writing activities.

An ergonomically correct posture in handwriting typically involves:

- Sitting with feet flat on the floor or supported by a footrest, knees at a right angle, and hips slightly higher than knees.
- Maintaining a straight back with shoulders relaxed and elbows close to the body.

- Positioning the writing surface at a height that allows the forearm to be parallel to the ground and the wrist to remain in a neutral position.
- Ensuring adequate lighting and proper distance between the eyes and the writing surface to reduce eye strain.

7. VISUAL SCANNING SKILLS

Visual scanning skills in handwriting refer to the ability to move the eyes efficiently and accurately across written text to gather information, identify letters, words, and punctuation marks, and interpret their meaning. It involves systematic and organized eye movements, such as left-to-right scanning in languages that read from left to right, or top-to-bottom scanning in vertically-oriented scripts.

Effective visual scanning skills are essential for tasks such as reading, copying, and writing, as they enable individuals to locate specific information, track their progress, and identify errors. Deficits in visual scanning skills can lead to difficulties in handwriting, including illegibility, slow writing speed, and errors in letter formation and spacing.

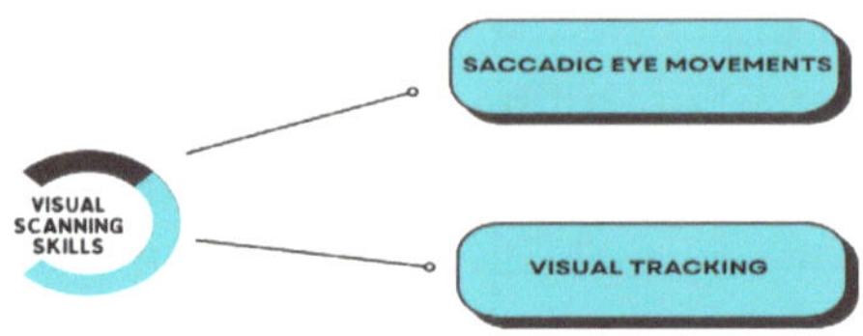

Saccadic Eye Movements

Saccadic eye movements in handwriting refer to rapid and coordinated movements of the eyes as they shift from one fixation point to another during the act of writing. These movements involve quick, jerky motions that allow individuals to efficiently scan and gather visual information from their surroundings. In the context of handwriting, saccadic eye movements help guide the eyes along the lines of text being read or written, enabling the brain to process and interpret the visual input.

Visual Tracking

Visual tracking in handwriting refers to the ability to follow a moving object or visual stimuli smoothly and accurately with the eyes, particularly in the context of reading and writing. It involves coordinating eye movements to track the motion of the writing instrument as it moves across the page during the act of writing or to follow the progression of text while reading. Efficient visual tracking skills are crucial for maintaining proper alignment, spacing, and legibility in handwriting, as well as for comprehending written material.

8. PERSISTENCE AND PATIENCE

Persistence and patience in handwriting refer to the ability to maintain effort and concentration over time, as well as the willingness to continue practicing and refining handwriting skills despite challenges or setbacks. It involves demonstrating resilience, determination, and a positive attitude toward improving handwriting abilities.

Individuals who exhibit persistence and patience in handwriting are more likely to engage in regular practice, seek out assistance when needed, and persevere through difficulties to achieve their handwriting goals. These qualities are essential for overcoming obstacles, building confidence, and ultimately achieving success in handwriting tasks.

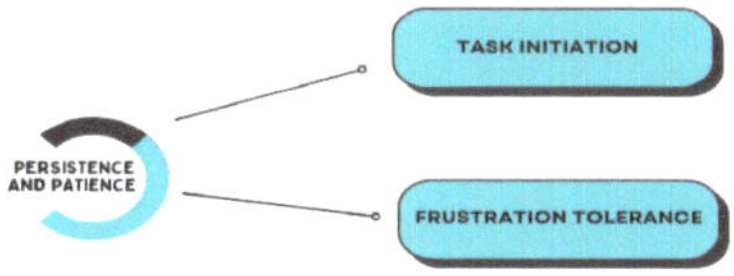

Task Initiation

Task initiation in handwriting refers to the ability to begin a writing-related activity promptly and independently. It involves overcoming procrastination or hesitation and starting the writing task with focus and determination. Individuals who demonstrate strong task initiation skills in handwriting can set goals, prioritize tasks, and initiate the writing process effectively without undue delay.

Frustration Tolerance

Frustration tolerance in handwriting refers to an individuals ability to manage and cope with feelings of frustration, annoyance, or disappointment that may arise during the writing process. It involves maintaining composure, staying focused, and persisting in the task despite encountering difficulties such as making mistakes, experiencing hand fatigue, or encountering challenges with letter formation or spacing.

Individuals with strong frustration tolerance in handwriting can effectively regulate their emotions, maintain a positive attitude, and continue working towards their writing goals without becoming overwhelmed or discouraged by setbacks.

OCCUPATIONAL THERAPY ROLE IN FAR-POINT COPYING

Occupational Therapy plays a significant role in far-point copying handwriting tasks, especially for individuals with difficulties such as dysgraphia or fine motor challenges. In far-point copying, individuals are required to copy written material from a distant source, such as a chalkboard or a distant text, onto their own paper. This task requires coordination of visual perception, visual-motor integration, fine motor skills, and attention.

Occupational Therapists can intervene in far-point coping handwriting tasks through various strategies:

- **Visual perception and visual-motor integration training**: Occupational Therapists can provide exercises and activities to improve visual perception skills, such as visual discrimination, figure-ground perception, and visual memory. Additionally, they can implement interventions to enhance visual-motor integration, ensuring that individuals can accurately copy visual information onto paper.
- **Fine motor skill development**: Occupational Therapists can utilize activities and exercises to enhance fine motor skills, including hand strength, dexterity, and finger coordination. Strengthening these skills can improve the precision and control needed for handwriting tasks, including far-point copying.
- **Adaptive equipment and environmental modifications**: Occupational Therapists can recommend and provide adaptive equipment such as slant boards, magnifying tools, or specialized writing implements to facilitate far-point copying tasks. They may also suggest environmental modifications, such as adjusting lighting or seating arrangements, to optimize the individual's performance during copying tasks.
- **Sensory integration techniques**: For individuals with sensory processing difficulties, Occupational Therapists can implement sensory integration techniques to address sensory sensitivities or sensory-seeking behaviors that may impact far-point coping handwriting tasks. By addressing sensory needs, individuals can better focus and engage in the task at hand.

OCCUPATIONAL THERAPY INTERVENTION FOR FAR-POINT COPYING

Occupational Therapists often draw from a variety of sources and evidence-based practices to design interventions. However, here are some examples of activities commonly used in Occupational Therapy practice for addressing far-point copying skills:

Visual Scanning Activities: Activities such as puzzles, hidden picture games, or search-and-find books can help improve visual scanning abilities, which are essential for locating and copying information from a distance.

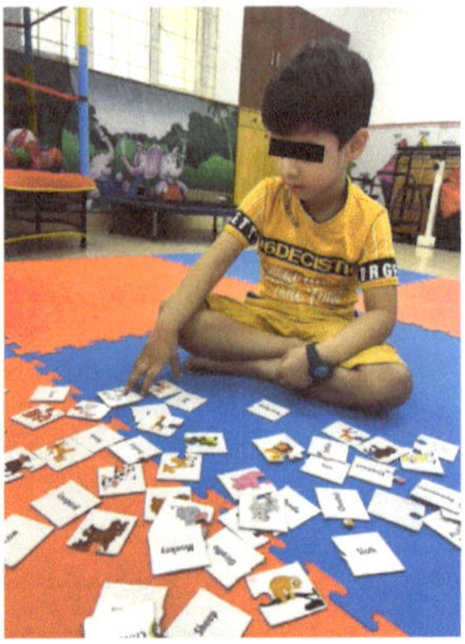

Activities included:

- Word search puzzles
- Find the difference
- Copycat drawing
- Visual tracking worksheets
- Memory games
- Alphabet scavenger hunt
- Visual discrimination sorting
- Interactive whiteboard games
- Magnified copying
- Obstacle course navigation
- Visual attention cards
- Directional games
- Hidden picture worksheets
- Digital interactive games
- Board games
- Book Reading
- Maze Game

Visual-Motor Integration Tasks: Tasks like tracing mazes, connecting dots to form shapes or letters, or copying geometric designs from a distance can enhance visual-motor coordination necessary for far-point copying.

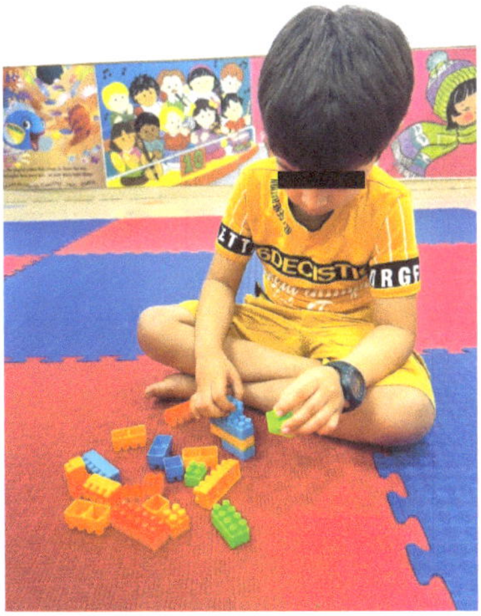

Activities included:

- Dot-to-dot drawing
- Tracing shapes and patterns
- Handwriting practice
- Coloring activities
- Cutting and pasting
- Stringing beads or lacing cards
- Puzzle play
- Drawing with chalk or sidewalk paint
- Threading activities
- Building with blocks

Use of Visual Aids: Therapists may utilize tools like magnifiers, slant boards, or specialized glasses to assist individuals with visual perception difficulties in far-point copying tasks.

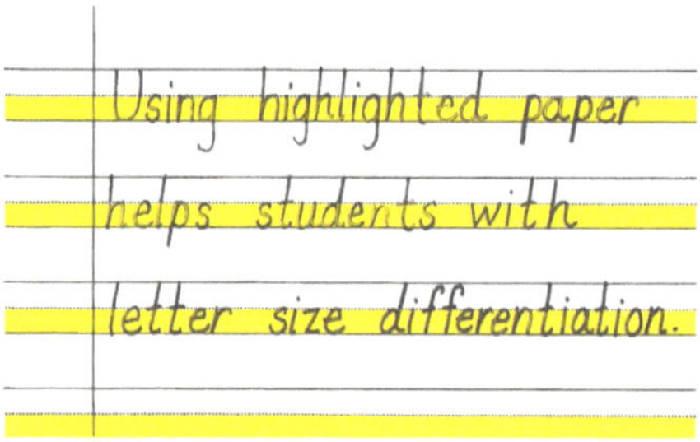

Activities included:

- Highlighted paper
- Magnifying glass
- Slant board
- Visual models
- Visual timers
- Highlighted text
- Visual prompts
- Large print materials

Gradual Distance Copying: Therapists can start individuals with copying tasks at a closer distance and gradually increase the distance as their skills improve, helping them to adapt to the demands of far-point copying gradually.

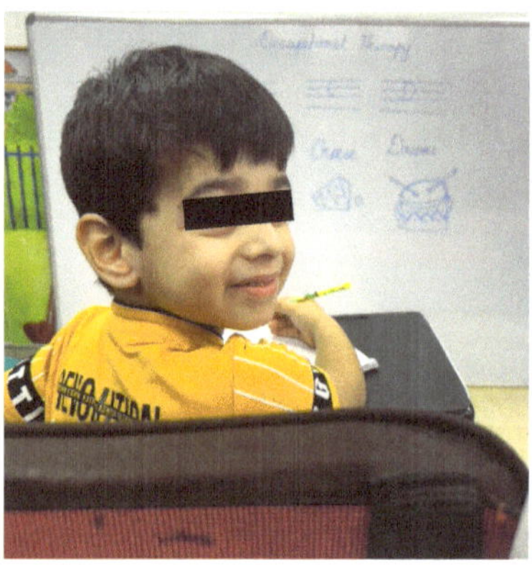

Activities included:

- Progressive letter copying
- Word wall copying
- Visual model copying
- Sentence strip copying
- Interactive whiteboard copying
- Guided copying activities
- Partner copying
- Timed copying challenges
- Obstacle course copying
- Outdoor copying activities

Technology-Assisted Activities: Interactive whiteboards, computer software, or apps designed for visual-motor integration tasks can provide engaging opportunities for practicing far-point copying skills in a controlled setting.

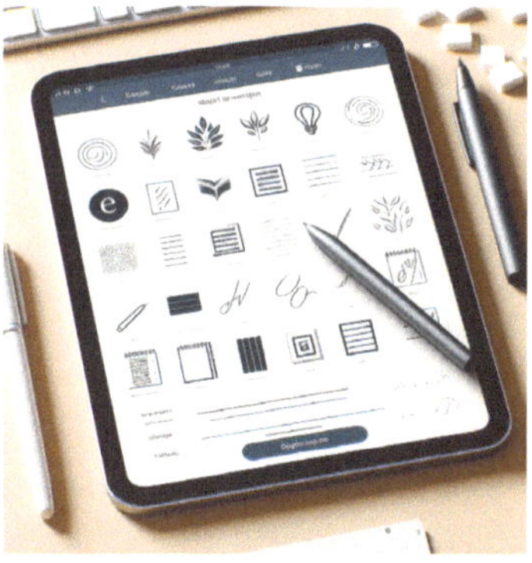

Activities included:

- Digital worksheets
- Online copying games
- Digital magnifiers
- Online handwriting platform

Multi-Sensory Approaches: Incorporating tactile materials, auditory cues, or kinesthetic elements into copying tasks can engage multiple senses and reinforce learning for individuals with diverse learning styles or sensory preferences.

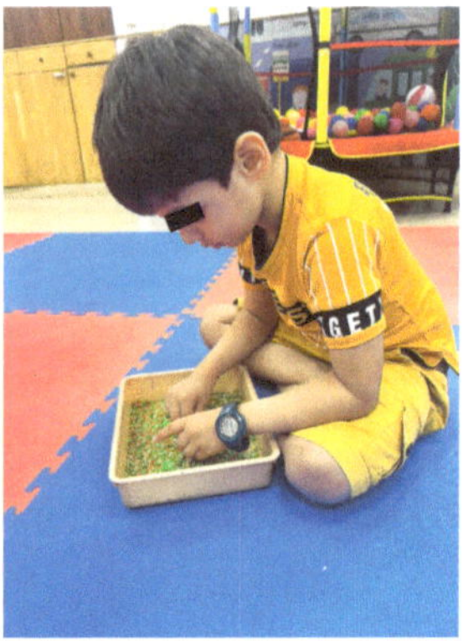

Activities included:

- Sandpaper letters
- Kinetic sand tracing
- Gel boards
- Visual-motor stations
- Scented markers or pens
- Sensory fine motor tools

Environmental Modifications: Therapists may suggest adjustments to the environment, such as optimizing lighting conditions or minimizing visual distractions, to support individuals during far-point copying activities.

Environmental modification includes

- Optimal lighting
- Contrast
- Positioning
- Ergonomic seating

- Workspace organization
- Quiet environment
- Visual aids
- Sensory supports
- Accessibility features

SUMMARY

Far point copying is a visual-motor skill where individuals accurately replicate letters, shapes, or images from a distance onto paper. It is crucial for early childhood development, aiding in motor skill development, reading, and visual arts. Skills required for far point copying include visual perception, visual-motor integration, fine motor control, and attention to detail. Occupational Therapists play a vital role in improving far point copying through interventions like visual scanning exercises, visual-motor integration tasks, use of visual aids, gradual distance copying, technology-assisted activities, multisensory approaches, and environmental modifications. These interventions aim to enhance skills such as visual perception, fine motor control, attention, and patience, supporting individuals in achieving handwriting proficiency and academic success.

ACCOMMODATIONS AND MODIFICATIONS FOR HANDWRITING PROBLEMS

WRITING AIDS:

- **Pencil grips:** To improve grip and control.
- **Weighted pens:** To help with motor control.
- **Slant boards:** To provide an optimal writing angle.
- **Special paper:** With raised lines or highlighted margins for better guidance.

ENVIRONMENTAL ADJUSTMENTS:

- **Comfortable seating:** Ensure the individual has an ergonomic chair and desk setup.
- **Proper lighting:** Adequate lighting to reduce eye strain and improve focus.
- **Quiet environment:** Minimize distractions to help the individual concentrate.

INSTRUCTIONAL STRATEGIES:

- **Multi-sensory techniques:** Use tactile, visual, and auditory methods to teach writing.
- **Step-by-step instructions:** Break down tasks into smaller, manageable steps.
- **Modeling:** Demonstrate proper handwriting techniques.
- Frequent breaks: Allow short breaks to prevent fatigue and maintain focus.

PRACTICE AND REINFORCEMENT:

- **Regular practice:** Short, consistent practice sessions to build muscle memory.
- **Positive reinforcement:** Encourage and praise efforts and improvements.
- **Interactive games:** Use games and activities that promote fine motor skills.

ACCOMMODATIONS IN ACADEMIC SETTINGS:

- **Extended time:** Allow extra time for writing tasks and exams.
- **Scribes:** Provide a scribe to write down the individual's verbal responses.
- **Flexible deadlines:** Offer flexibility with deadlines for written assignments.
- **Reduced writing load:** Modify assignments to reduce the amount of writing required.

ERGONOMIC ADJUSTMENTS:

- **Proper seating:** Ensure the child is seated properly with feet flat on the floor, hips, and knees at 90-degree angles.
- **Correct paper positioning:** Angle the paper appropriately (usually about 30 degrees for right-handed writers, and the opposite angle for left-handed writers) to facilitate better wrist and hand movement.
- **Writing surface:** Use a slanted desk or writing board to help with posture and writing angle.

PAPER MODIFICATIONS:

- **Lined paper:** Use paper with bold lines or raised lines to help with letter placement.
- **Graph paper:** This can assist with spatial organization and letter sizing.

- **Highlighting:** Highlight the writing area or use different colors to guide writing.

PRE-WRITING ACTIVITIES:

- **Fine motor exercises:** Engage in activities that strengthen the hand muscles such as squeezing stress balls, using clothespins, or playing with clay.
- **Finger aerobics:** Finger tapping, spreading fingers wide, and making different hand shapes can enhance dexterity.
- **Tracing shapes:** Practice tracing different shapes and patterns to develop control.

WRITING PRACTICE:

- **Letter formation:** Use multi-sensory approaches like tracing letters in sand, forming letters with clay, or using apps designed for handwriting practice.
- **Copying and tracing:** Start with tracing letters and then progress to copying letters, words, and sentences.
- **Slow and steady:** Encourage writing slowly and focusing on each letter's formation rather than speed.

TECHNOLOGY AIDS:

- **Typing:** Teach typing skills as an alternative for children who struggle significantly with handwriting.
- **Speech-to-text Software:** Use software that converts spoken words into text.
- **Digital tablets:** Tablets with styluses can provide an engaging way to practice handwriting.

COGNITIVE AND PERCEPTUAL STRATEGIES:

- **Visual cues:** Use visual guides and prompts for letter formation and placement.

- **Memory aids:** Use mnemonics or songs to help remember the steps in forming letters.
- **Consistent Practice:** Regular, short practice sessions are more effective than occasional long sessions.

CLASSROOM ACCOMMODATIONS:

- **Extended time:** Provide additional time for writing assignments.
- **Alternative assignments:** Allow oral reports or typed assignments when appropriate.
- **Reduced writing load:** Shorten the length of writing assignments or break them into smaller, manageable tasks.

HOME PROGRAM-AN OCCUPATIONAL THERAPISTS' PERSPECTIVE

A Home program in Occupational Therapy refers to a personalized set of activities prescribed by an Occupational Therapist for a patient to perform independently at home. These programs were designed to help individuals enhance their functional abilities and manage daily activities more effectively.

Here are some key components typically included in a home program in Occupational Therapy:

1. Initial Assessment.
2. Goal setting.
3. Activity selection.
4. Instruction and training
5. Adaptations and modifications
6. Progress tracking.
7. Reassessment.
8. Adjusting goals and activities.

IMPORTANCE OF HOME PROGRAM:

An Occupational Therapy home program for handwriting is crucial for a variety of reasons. It provides consistent, individualized, and practical techniques that can significantly improve a person's handwriting skills.

Here are significant points highlighting the importance of such programs:

1. **Consistency and Repetition:** Handwriting improvement requires regular practice. A home program requires regular or frequent handwriting practice, which helps reinforce skills learned during therapy sessions.
2. **Individualized attention:** Home programs are customized to individualized personal needs and concerns, providing targeted activities and strategies that directly benefit their unique handwriting issues.
3. **Comprehensive skill development**: Handwriting is not just about forming letters; it involves fine motor skills, eye - hand coordination, visual-motor integration, and cognitive skills. A home program addresses all these areas, promoting overall development.
4. **Parental Involvement:** Parents and caregivers play an active role in the therapy process, learning how to support and encourage the individual. This collaboration enhances the effectiveness of the interventions.
5. **Monitoring Progress:** Regular home program practice allows for continuous monitoring of progress. Therapists can perform assessment periodically and adjust the program as needed to keep it effective and challenging.
6. **Empowering Independence**: Improving handwriting skills at home builds confidence in one's abilities. This empowerment fosters greater independence in academic, occupational, and daily tasks.

RECORDING HOME PROGRAMS:

Recording home programs in Occupational Therapy is essential for tracking progress, monitoring adherence, and adjusting interventions as necessary. Home program can be properly documented using a variety of charts and forms.

Here are some common charts used to record home programs:

1. **Daily Activity Log:** This chart allows individuals or caregivers to record the completion of home program activities on a daily basis.
2. **Goal tracking charts:** It help individuals and therapists in identifying milestones and adjusting interventions accordingly.
3. **Rating Scales or Likert Scales:** These tools involve to analyse the individual's performance, progress, or perceived difficulty of home program activities.
4. **Weekly or Monthly Progress Summary:** It provides a summary of the individual's participation, progress, and challenges encountered during the home program.
5. **Outcome Measures or Assessments:** It is used to evaluate the effectiveness of the home program and track changes in functional abilities over time.

HOME PROGRAM SHEET:

S.No	Name of the Activity	Schedule Checklist	Repetition	Adaptation	Gradation
01.					

INTERVENTION / ACTIVITY RECORDING SHEET:

Date	Intervention / Activity	Task Completion	Feedback of Parents/ caregivers	Need for the Change

GOALS SHEET - HOME PROGRAM TIMELINE – ATTENDANCE SCHEDULE:

S.No	Day	Activity Completion Status	Meltdowns	Reinforcements
01	Monday			
02	Tuesday			
03	Wednesday			
04	Thursday			
05	Friday			
06	Saturday			
07	Sunday			

Weekly goal achievements:

Parents feedback:

Goals for the next week:

Therapist suggestion:

HOME PROGRAM ACTIVITIES FOR FINE & GROSS MOTOR SKILLS IN RELATION TO HANDWRITING:

GROSS MOTOR ACTIVITIES:

1. Jumping jacks
2. Indoor yoga
3. Hide and seek
4. Push-ups
5. Indoor parade
6. Blanket tug-of-war
7. Hopscotch
8. Obstacle course

9. Scrub floors with soapy water
10. Dancing
11. Crawl through tunnels
12. Marching games
13. Wash walls
14. Walking on the pillows
15. Walking on the sleeping eight
16. Ball throwing and catching
17. Bowling
18. Skipping
19. Animal walk
20. Target kicking

FINE MOTOR ACTIVITIES:

1. Making letters using Clay.
2. Playing with tweezers to pick up beads or small objects.
3. Coloring activity.
4. Cutting with safety scissors.
5. Play dough.
6. Coin drop in piggy bank.
7. Stringing beads.
8. Sand play.
9. Vegetable painting.
10. Collage.
11. Finger Painting.
12. Hanging cloth clips.
13. Lacing activity.
14. Nuts and Bolts activity.
15. Matching and sorting activities.
16. Art and crafts.
17. Ripping and crumbling papers.
18. Maze activity.
19. Putting pegs into pegboard.
20. Necklace using Pasta.

WARM-UP ACTIVITIES TO PRACTICE HAND WRITING SKILL AT HOME:

1. Press down hard on desktop with both hands.
2. Briskly rub hands together.
3. Place the fingertips together and do finger "push-ups".
4. Pass around a weighted ball.
5. Stretch thick rubber bands between fingers and thumb.
6. Squeeze hands into fist.

GENERAL HANDWRITING ASSESSMENT FORM

Name of the Client:	

Age / Gender:

Date of Birth:

Date of Assessment:

Class / Grade:

Examiner:

Before starting the assessment, make sure that the table and chair are positioned correctly.

PRE - REQUISITE COMPONENT	YES/ NO
Feet flat on the floor, upright, lower back is supported by the chair.	
Desk height and writing surface is at or slightly above the elbow crease.	
Stabilizes paper with nondominant hand.	
Holds pencil with appropriate tripod grasp.	
Demonstrates hand dominance.	
Ability to cross mid-line of the body.	
Pencil pressure appropriate – not too heavy or light.	
Maintains appropriate grasp with adequate strength throughout the duration of the activity	
COMMENT:	

PRE-WRITING SKILLS	YES / NO
Can draw horizontal and vertical lines.	
Can combine horizontal and vertical lines.	
Can draw shapes.	
Can be able to do coloring activity.	
COMMENT:	

FINE MOTOR SKILLS	YES / NO
Moves an object from palm to finger or finger to palm.	
Turns pencil around to erase the mistake without assistance from the other hand or another surface.	
Can demonstrate adequate control of the writing tool (dot to dot or maze activity).	
COMMENT:	

PRESENTATION AND SPACING:	YES / NO
Proper position of words on the line.	
Consistent letter size.	
Consistent spacing between the words.	
Are the words or letters floating.	
Are letters joined correctly.	
Starts on the left side margin of the page.	
Reversal of letters.	
Mixture of upper- and lower-case letters.	
COMMENT:	

VISUAL PERCEPTUAL COMPONENTS:	YES / NO
Recognizes strokes, numbers and letters.	
Stays within the boundary for coloring and writing.	
Copies entire word or line with single glance.	
COMMENT:	

SENSORY PROCESSING COMPONENT:	YES / NO
Completes task independently or with minimal cues.	
Complete task within the time.	
Knows to differentiate right from left and top from down.	
COMMENT:	

VISUO-MOTOR COMPONENTS:	YES / NO
Can able to imitate basic strokes and shapes.	
Can able to draw recognizable pictures.	
Copies basic strokes, numbers, letters, shapes and pictures from near point.	
Copies basic strokes, numbers, letters, shapes and pictures from far point.	
COMMENT:	

HANDWRITING CHECKLIST	YES/NO
Did I write each and every letter clearly in order for someone else to read it?	
Did I use a consistent letter size throughout my writing (i.e., short letters were short and tall letters were tall)?	
Did I write all the letters with proper spacing?	
Did I write all the letters on the line?	
Did I erase my mistakes rather than over writing it?	
Is my writing being fluent?	

While a general assessment can provide valuable insights into a person's handwriting abilities, for more comprehensive and standardized evaluation, particularly for therapeutic purposes, it's recommended to involve an Occupational Therapist. Occupational Therapists have specialized training in assessing and addressing handwriting difficulties, using standardized scales and techniques to tailor interventions to individual needs. They can provide targeted interventions and strategies to improve handwriting skills and overcome challenges.

HANDWRITING WORKSHEETS

SAMPLE

Scribble to script

Manuscript

ABCDEFGHIJKLMNOPQRSTUVWXYZ

Cursive

Abcdefghijklmnopqrstuvwxyz

SAMPLE WORKSHEETS

Right Hander's

Left Hander's

COLOURING WORKSHEETS

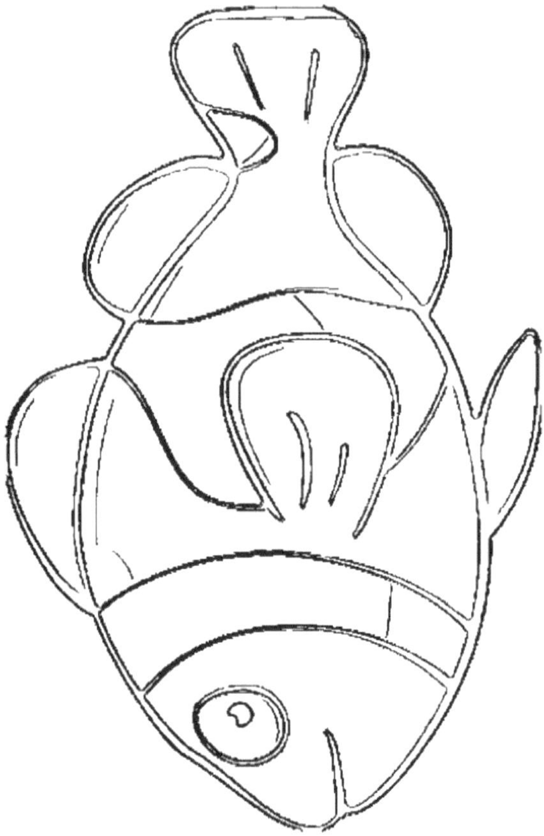

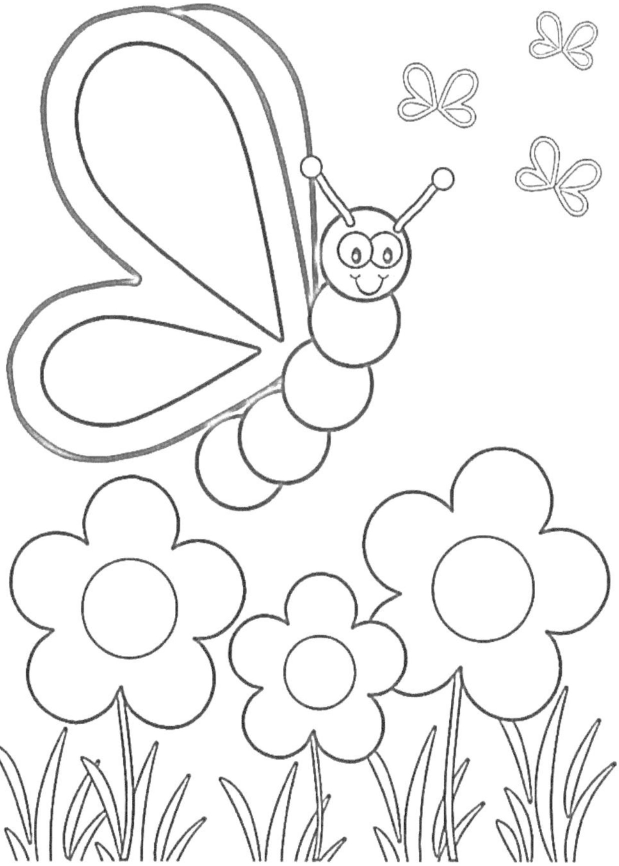

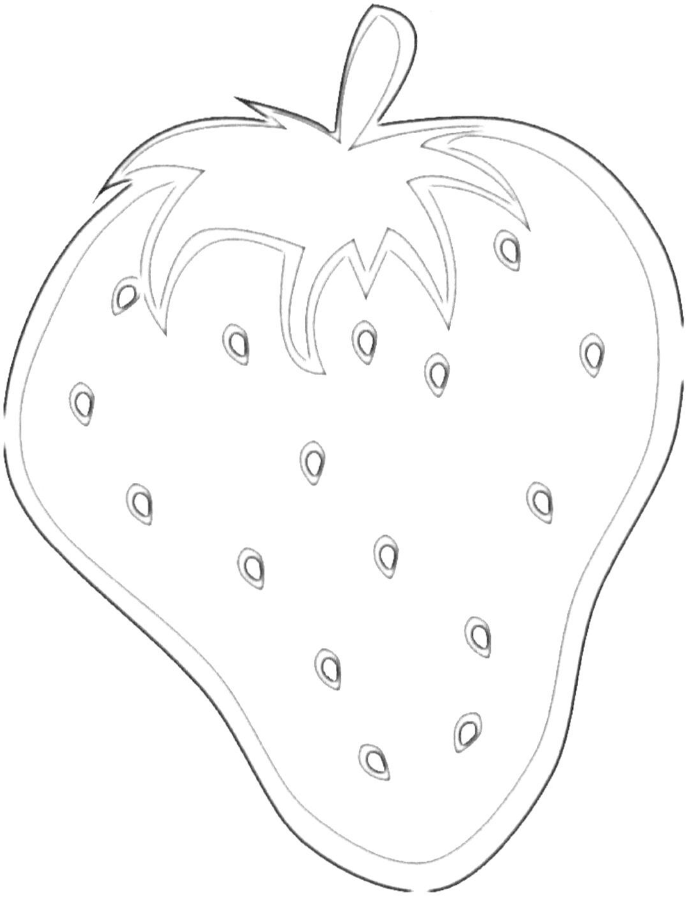

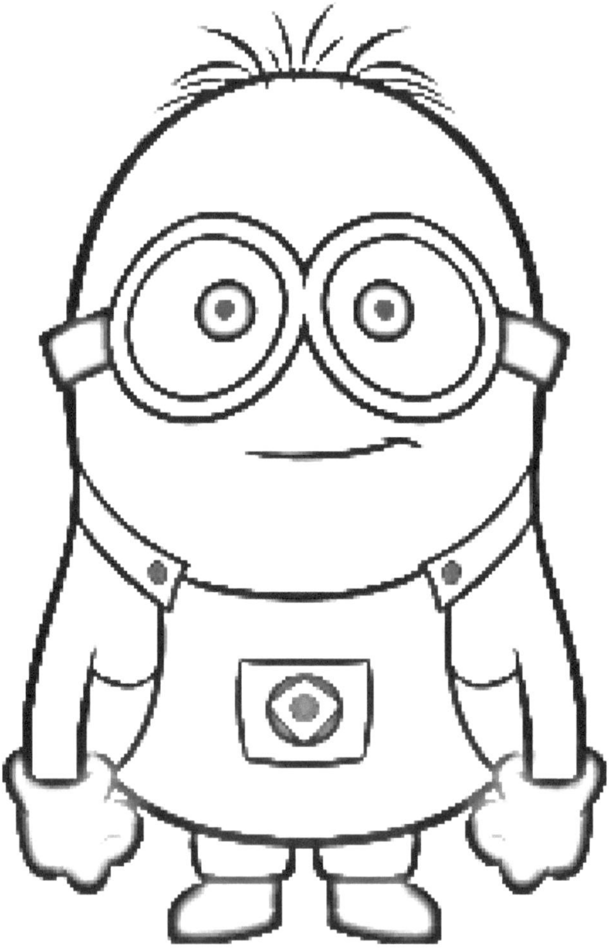

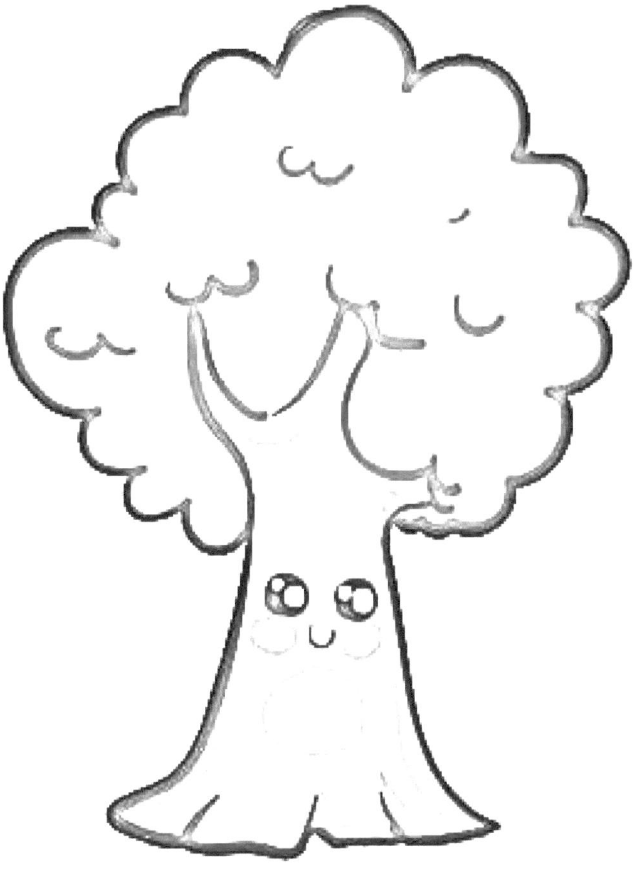

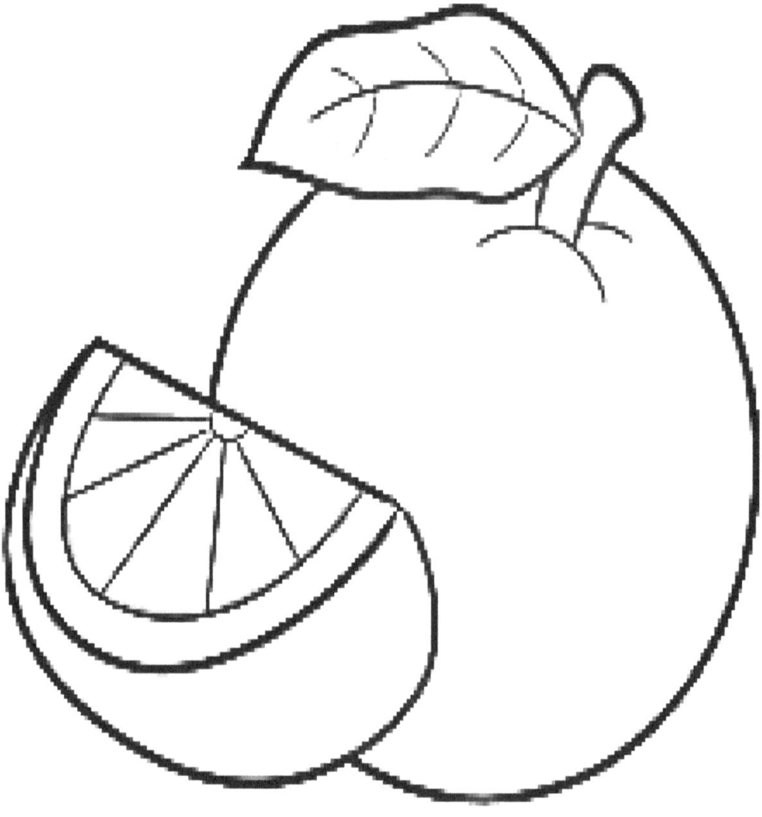

Basic strokes

Example 1:

Example 2: cccccccccccccccccccccccccccccccc

Example 3: nnnnnnnnnnnnnnnn

Example 4: uuuuuuuuu

Example 5: sssssssssssssssssssssssss

Example 6:

Example 7: mmmmmmmmmmmmmm...

Alphabets

Example 1:

A B C D E F G H I J K L M...
N O P Q R S T U V W X Y Z

Example 2:

A B C D E F G H I J K L M

N O P Q R S T U V W X Y Z

Example 3:

a b c d e f g h i j k l m

n o p q r s t u v w x y z

Example 4: lllffffllllffffllllffffllllffffllllffffllllffff

Example 5: *eeehhhheeeehhhheeeehhhheeeehhhh*

Example 6: *ekhekhekhekhekhekhekhekhekhekh*

Example 7: felfelfelfelfelfelfelfelfelfelfelfelfelfelfelfelfel

Stretches & Speed drills

Example 1:...

age age age age age age age age age age

age age age age age age age age age

Example 2:...

edge edge edge edge edge edge edge edge

edge edge edge edge edge edge edge edge

Example 3:

like like like like like like like like like

like like like like like like like like like like

Example 4:

back back back back back back back

back back back back back back back back

Range control
&
Stretches

Example 1:

Example 2: 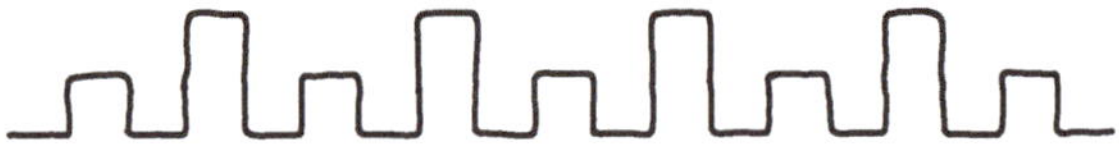

Example 3:

Monday

Monday

Tuesday

Tuesday

Wednesday

Wednesday

Thursday

Thursday

Friday

Friday

Saturday

Saturday

Sunday

Sunday

Example 4:

January...

January

February

February

March

March

April

April

May

May

June

June

July

July

August

August...

September

September

October

October

November

November

December

December

Carbon copy

Example 1:...

I can write

I can write...

Example 2:

You can read this

You can read this

Example 3:

Animals cannot cook

Animals cannot cook...

Example 4:...

Jack just got a jar

Jack just got a jar

Example 5:

Uma is under the umbrella

Uma is under the umbrella

Example 6:

Ben saw Julie at the zoo

Ben saw Julie at the zoo...

Example 7:

Hockey is India's National sport

Hockey is India's National sport

Endurance Training

Example 1:

Wake up early and go to bed early

Wake up early and go to bed early...

Example 2:...

Always wash fruits and vegetables before cooking

Always wash fruits and vegetables before cooking

Example 3:

Write about yourself in a paragraph

Write about yourself in a paragraph

Example 4:

Write about the most used things in a classroom

Write about the most used things in a classroom

Example 5:

Write a letter to your friend

Write a letter to your friend...

Example 5:

Write a paragraph of 50 words

Write a paragraph of 50 words

Good work

Congratulations

www.ingramcontent.com/pod-product-compliance
Ingram Content Group UK Ltd.
Pitfield, Milton Keynes, MK11 3LW, UK
UKHW061030310726
14089UKWH00007B/167
9798894463193